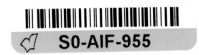

Supervision in Health Care Organizations

BOOKS OF RELATED INTEREST

McFarland/Leonard/Morris: *Nursing Leadership and Management: Contemporary Strategies,* 1983, 0-471-09097-2

Schweiger: *The Nurse as Manager,* 1980, 0-471-04343-5

SUPERVISION IN HEALTH CARE ORGANIZATIONS

RICHARD I. LYLES, Ph.D.
Principal
Situation Management Systems, Inc.
Plymouth, Massachusetts
R. I. Lyles and Associates, Inc.
Poway, California

CARL JOINER, Ph.D.
Associate Professor
School of Business
Mercer University
Macon, Georgia

A Wiley Medical Publication
John Wiley & Sons
New York • Chichester • Brisbane • Toronto • Singapore

Library of Congress Cataloging in Publication Data:

Lyles, Richard I.
  Supervision in health care organizations.

  (A Wiley medical publication)
  Includes bibliographies and index.
  1. Nursing service administration.   2. Supervision
of employees.   I. Joiner, Carl.   II. Title.
III. Series.   [DNLM: 1. Administrative Personnel.
2. Delivery of Health Care—organization & administration.   3. Personnel Management. W 88 L985s]
RT89.L95   1986   362.1'1'068   85-17799
ISBN 0-471-80459-2

Printed in the United States of America

10 9 8 7 6 5 4 3 2 1

To our families, with love

Foreword

The health care "field" is rapidly becoming a health care "industry." (The field is not yet organizationally sophisticated enough to be called an industry nor "connected" enough to be called a system.) And events are beginning to form trends that should interest readers of this exceptionally timely book.

With increasing energy, health care organizations across the country are devoting larger shares of their resources to become competitive, to develop strategies, and to build management structures and systems—in short, to survive. The health care field is developing, organizationally, similar to the way the food industry evolved during the 1950s, 1960s, and 1970s, but at an unparalleled pace. The corner grocery (solo practitioner) becomes the supermarket (group practice). The independent supermarket (community hospital with outpatient departments) becomes Safeway (Hospital Corporation of America, American Medical International). But while we are racing toward an industry, we are only beginning to crawl toward a rational, coherent, connected health care system.

The *field* has been criticized for being too costly, too inefficient, ineffective, and unresponsive to its customers. Customers (patients, corporations, and government) blame physicians; physicians blame insurance companies, government, and lawyers; nurses blame physicians and allied health professionals; allied health professionals blame physicians, nurses, and other allied health professionals; and administrators blame everybody. But blaming has produced no rewards for anyone. Criticism of the health care field, however, is still warranted. But in my opinion, the criticism has been directed at everything except the fundamental problem—namely, the field is seriously undermanaged.

Current management practices in the health care field would not be acceptable in private industry or in the future health care industry. Qualitatively, we are 10 to 20 years behind private industry. Quantitatively, we have less than half the trained managers and supervisors needed for the highly complex organizations characterizing the health care field. (These observations are not intended as an attack on health care administrators. The field, until recently, viewed management as "overhead," provided few rewards for its managers, and had little incentive to develop better management.)

The most glaring deficiency in the health care field is management; more precisely, the depth of management among the supervisors of those who actually produce the work: in essence, nurses, allied health professionals, physicians, psychologists, and social workers. Too little time, effort, and money are devoted to developing these critical supervisors and managers. The result is typically an organization laden with executives, administrators, middle managers, secretaries, and clerks in the business or administrative departments, and a token or laissez-faire approach to the management and supervision of the production departments (i.e., physicians, nurses, allied health professionals). This condition is tolerable in the health care "field," but will become intolerable for the health care "industry."

The question is not whether the health care industries will demand better management for its physicians, nurses, and allied health professionals, but *who* can provide the best management and supervision of these professionals. Many will argue that professional managers (MBAs, MHAs) are best suited for the role. But one need only review the classic article by Victor Vroom, "A New Look at Managerial Decision Making," to see why hospitals, group practices, HMOs, and other organizations in the health care field are not following that argument. According to Vroom, "acceptance" of a decision by those who must implement it is critical for an effective decision. And "acceptance" of the manager or supervisor by allied health professionals, nurses, and physicians is primarily determined by whether "he or she understands my work, my skills, my ethics." Consequently, for example, nurses are more likely to "accept" another nurse and his or her decisions than a nonnurse and his or her decisions, *even though* the decisions made by each are qualitatively identical. The same is true, I believe, for allied health professionals and physicians. However, I hasten to add that nurses, allied health professionals, or physicians who make "bad" managerial decisions will lose their "acceptance" or credibility as fast, if not faster, than a nonclinician, because it cannot be said that they did not understand the nature of the work.

From my perspective, the trend is clear—an increasing number of "white coats" will enter managerial and supervisory positions. This trend will be driven by two conditions. Nurses, allied health professionals, and physicians are and will increasingly seek, for a wide variety of personal decisions, new challenges, opportunities, and rewards outside their parent professions. Second, because of the current over-capacity of patient care, "white coat" jobs will be reduced by competition and changes in payment status.

The real challenge to nurses and other health professionals moving into managerial and supervisory positions will, in my opinion, be the same as that confronting physicians—to make a clear and unqualified distinction between the clinical professions and the management professions. Nursing, as well as each of the allied health professions, has its own body of knowledge, language, skills, and ethics, and so does the profession of management. Nurses and allied health professionals are "doers." They do "the work"—the patient care, the lab work, the radiology work—the principle work that the provider organization has been established to do.

Managers and supervisors do not do "the work." Managers and supervisors are designers or architects. Their primary responsibility is to help design ways so that the "doers" can do their work quicker, more efficiently, more effectively, or better. One real problem for "white coats" moving into "suit coat" roles is carrying their "doer" behaviors into designer roles.

Learning the language of the managerial and supervisory professions is another challenge to nurses, allied health professionals, and physicians aspiring to leadership roles. Credibility in these roles must be established not only with the "doers," but also with other management and supervisory professionals. One test other managers will apply to the "white coat" manager or supervisor is the "fluency test." Do you speak *our* language? You are on our turf now and here we speak "management." It is difficult to be credible in any profession if one does not speak the language of that profession.

Rewards for nurses and allied health professionals are quite different from those of managers and supervisors. "White coat" rewards tend to be more immediate and personal or intimate. Rewards for managers and supervisors are more long-term and vicarious. The loss of the immediate personal gratification of patient care is probably the most significant stressor for "white coats" who become "suit coats."

But although there are some significant traps, challenges, and stressors for physicians, nurses, and allied health professionals in becoming managers and supervisors, the rewards, in my opinion, tip the scales. The "white coat" carries the glass of water to the patient; the manager builds the aqueduct. If you choose to build aqueducts in the evolving health care industry, the authors of this text have provided the tools.

ROGER S. SCHENKE
American Academy of Medical Directors
American College of Physician Executives
Orlando, Florida

Preface

More than 4.3 million people are currently employed in more than 60,000 organizations that deliver health care in the United States. These numbers are increasing steadily. The U.S. Labor Department predicts this increase will continue into the twenty-first century.

Health care specialists, through the organizations in which they work, provide a service that is becoming increasingly more complex. Efficient delivery relies on the effective coordination of people who possess diverse skills and expertise. The burden of this coordination activity is falling increasingly onto the shoulders of nurses and allied health professionals who, after having performed well in their area of professional expertise, have been promoted into the supervisory ranks.

This basic text presents the fundamentals of supervision that a nurse or allied health professional will need in fulfilling positions of higher organizational responsibility. A definite distinction is made between the technical work of actually *providing* a specific service and *supervising* the work of others who are providing these specialized services.

It is our belief that the readers of this book are not interested in becoming management experts. Rather, our readers are more interested in learning the supervisory skills necessary to be able to achieve maximum satisfaction and rewards in their primary area of vocational pursuit—the field of health care. Accordingly, where a choice existed between emphasizing either the practical or the theoretical, we have given more attention to the practical applications at the expense of theory. For those readers who desire to delve deeper into any one of the concepts, a list of references is provided at the end of each chapter.

The goal of this book is to present the material in such a way that people can both learn from the logical, applications-oriented method, and use the book as a reference source in the future. Used in this way, the book will serve as a handbook or manual that the reader can rely on long after its initial reading.

The first part of the book examines the role of the health care supervisor. The second part discusses the functions of health care supervision: planning, organizing, directing, and controlling. The third part is dedicated to the primary skills a supervisor will need to fulfill the role successfully. These skills include communication, problem solving and decision making, managing groups, time management, managing change, and conflict management. In the final unit, two chapters discuss the issues of application of management principles and ethics.

This final section should be of particular interest to readers. The case incidents included in Chapter 12 cover a broad range of difficult supervisory dilemmas likely to be encountered in the health care field. The discussion questions following each case will help focus the reader on the issues most important for each case. Not only should this help in understanding the material presented in the earlier chapters, but it should also aid readers in developing the skills of anticipatory thinking. We consider this to be an essential set of skills for the high-pressured and fast-paced work environment in the health care field of the immediate future.

We would like to acknowledge the special contributions that Dr. M. Wayne Wilson has made to this book. He perceived the basic need for the book and conceived of its practical structure and focus. The chapter on time management is, for the most part, based on years of his research. Many of the ideas in other chapters also resulted from his thinking.

RICHARD I. LYLES
CARL JOINER

Contents

PART FOUR: SUPERVISION IN THE WORLD OF HEALTH CARE

Supervision
in Health Care
Organizations

PART ONE

THE HEALTH CARE SUPERVISOR'S ROLE AND RESPONSIBILITIES

Chapter One

The Role of Supervision in Health Care Organizations

The day of the country doctor (or even the family doctor) visiting homes to deliver health care services is gone. More than 7,000 hospitals, 23,000 long-term care facilities, 20,000 nursing and residential care homes, 5,000 other types of medical facilities, and 40,000 clinics and physician's offices throughout the country comprise the health care delivery system. Other types of organizations, such as labs and health service agencies, have increased in number and have become more important components of health care delivery.

In today's world of high technology and specialization, the delivery of health care services requires a diversity of highly specialized skills. This mix of skills can be provided only by groups of people; hence, the need for organizations.

Organizations can deliver better quality and a make complete combination of services than an individual health service could provide. Organizations can offer more specialties, and they can also encourage their members to pursue specialization. Organizations typically provide a broader resource base (here we refer not only to talent and human resources, but also to equipment, capital, and facilities). And finally, organizations provide greater flexibility by being able to mix and match the demands of this broad resource base to meet the needs of various situations that arise.

THE NEED FOR MANAGEMENT-ORIENTED SUPERVISION

But why is management needed? If all these specialists are so highly trained and competent in their fields, then why can't they simply do their jobs? What if people in the organization were hired solely on the basis of their expertise in their fields and then were allowed to do their jobs without interference or problems created by administrators and managers?

The answers to these questions have little to do either with our trust or with our confidence in people with specialized knowledge or expertise. It is an issue of practicality. Experience indicates that it is impossible to gather a group of people, no matter how qualified they are in their fields, and expect good results to evolve naturally to meet the needs of the organization. To paraphrase management expert Peter Drucker (1973), the only things that naturally evolve in organizations are friction, frustration, irritation, dissatisfaction, unhappiness, and malperformance. For anything else to develop, someone must do something to make it happen. This is the role of management—namely, causing the desired results to happen.

Every organization is different. The services, each organization provides, as well as the people or organizations receiving services or products, are unique. Consequently, policies and practices vary from organization to organization. What may be right in one situation may be wrong in another and vice versa. The challenge to management is in trying to discover the best way to operate in circumstances.

First, management must define the purpose of the organization. Different organizations have different purposes; moreover, organizations usually have purposes that differ from the individual purposes of the people who comprise the organization. Someone must take the initiative to first identify the purpose of the organization, and then ensure that the energies and activities of the people in the organization are channelled in directions that will enable these purposes to be accomplished.

Someone must determine what activities must be conducted and then ensure that they happen as planned. Someone must resolve disputes, coordinate work to avoid duplication, and strive for efficiency. Someone must look toward the future and be prepared to respond to future demands. The people who do all this work are the supervisors and administrators in management-oriented positions who are engaged in the work of managing the organization. What then is management?

MANAGEMENT WORK DEFINED

The work of management can be described in a number of different ways. One fairly common description, usually attributed to Mary Parker Follet, describes management as, "the art of getting things done through people" (Stoner, 1978, p. 7). This ties in closely with the more traditional definition of managers as people who are primarily responsible for the work of other people. But in more recent years, Peter F. Drucker, noted management theorist, has encouraged us to adopt a different focus when defining management work. Drucker states that the emphasis should be on the contribution managers make to the organization, rather than on the amount of responsibility or control they have (Drucker, 1973).

In other words, when talking about the work managers do, rather than referring to the supervisor of nurses (focus on control), Drucker would encourage us to refer to the *supervisor of nursing*. The emphasis on the function of nursing and the delivery of nursing services would cause us to interpret intuitively that supervisor's role in the context of function rather than power. In turn, this encourages us to think in terms of contribution as a primary emphasis rather than control.

This concept is often overlooked, especially among the ranks of first-line supervisors. In health care organizations the essence of the first-line supervisor's job is to direct the efforts of subordinates in accomplishing the organization's goals. *But far too often the emphasis is on the subordinate and not the goal.* This action results in the supervisor not taking initiative to contribute to the aims of the organization. The supervisor becomes a controller rather than a leader, which inevitably leads to lower than optimal contribution and performance.

Another important aspect in understanding the roles of supervisors and the work of management concerns the extent to which they still work within their functional specialties or professional expertise as opposed to fulfilling their managerial activities. Another management theorist and researcher, Louis A. Allen, has observed that, when given a choice between doing the work of management or doing the operating work associated with their functional specialty, most supervisors will choose to do the operating work (Morrisey, 1977). In essence, they become "super-operators," or "super-technicians," or "super-nurses," instead of supervisors. When this happens, the organization suffers.

Management work is the activity associated with the functions of planning, organizing, staffing, directing, and controlling the efforts of individuals and the use of other resources to achieve individual, group, or organizational purposes. Supervisors, managers, and administrators are the people who perform these activities in the organization. These management processes are carried out at every level in the organization, from the top administrative or executive-level positions, down through the ranks of middle management and first-line supervision, and at least to some extent, even into the ranks of individual workers. To best understand the role of supervisors, it is helpful to examine some of the differences in the focus of effort from top to bottom in health care organizations. Although the functions and processes are basically the same from top to bottom, the focus of effort and type of responsibility relative to the processes differ at different levels.

Table 1.1 presents a comparison between the focus of top management and first-line supervision for each of the five management functions. The general description of activities normally associated with the function is presented in the column on the left, with the focus of the top administrative and managerial levels listed in the middle column. The focus of first-line supervision is listed in the right-hand column.

Another comparison that is important, but not obvious from Table 1.1, is the amount of time spent in each of the functional areas at different levels in the organization. Because of the differences in focus, these times will vary. Figure 1.1 illustrates the differences in the percentage of time supervisors will typically spend in each of the functional areas.

Top management is primarily concerned with long-range, total organization issues. At this level, policy is defined and direction is set. Middle management works to integrate the broad range of functions necessary to achieve the goals and to coordinate information and decisions. First-line supervision then shoulders the burden of implementation.

As a result, top management is more concerned with planning, organizing, and

Table 1.1

Functions of Management: Comparison of Focus, Top versus First-Line Supervision

Function	Focus of Top Administration	Focus of Supervision
Planning		
Forecasting	Long range	Short range
Budgeting	Growth	Day-to-Day
Establishing objectives	Capital Procurement	Week-to-Week
Scheduling	Service Mix	Converting "What" to "how to"
Developing policies	Initiating	Activities lists
	Overall financial	Scheduling tasks and facilities
Organizing		
Designing the organization	Overall structure	Coordination of people, equipment, and supplies
Establishing work relationships	Establish lines of responsibility & authority	to accomplish results
Work flow	Determine line and staff relationships	More concerned with relationships between things
Delegating		and specific activities than with overall structure.
Staffing		
Hiring people	Develop personnel policies	Hiring good staff
Recruiting people	Provide total training system	Training and developing workers
Promotion	to support	Assessing staff needs
Training	Negotiating union contracts	
Development		
Directing		
Motivating	Model good behavior	Leading in such a way as to
Leading	Develop and promote a positive overall approach to leadership	create a positive climate in which workers operate with optimum efficiency
	Provide good image in the community	and professionalism
Controlling		
Establishing standards	Monitor total organizational results	Tracking work in progress
Measuring, evaluating, and correcting performance	Set standards & goals	Appraising work and results Correcting performance

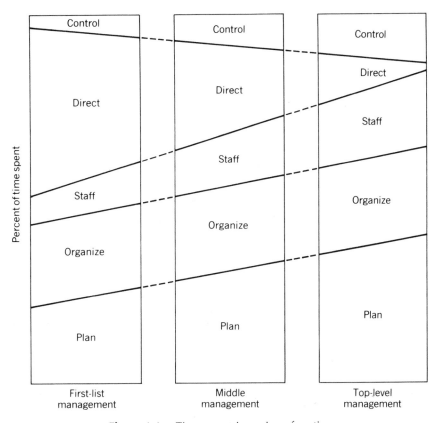

Figure 1.1. Time spent in various functions.

controlling, while supervisors are more concerned with staffing and directing. People at the top will naturally be drawn toward organizational issues, while supervisors will naturally focus more on individual issues. *A mistake many new supervisors make is in not realizing that it is primarily their responsibility and not that of top management to solve individual problems and to look after the individual needs of the workers.*

The supervisor, therefore, is in a unique position in the organization. The responsibilities are significant and the role is complex. Workers, for example, will turn to the supervisor to satisfy certain needs. Management will do the same for different needs. And patients and other service recipients will have still different needs. Some of the needs a supervisor in health care organizations will be expected to provide include the following:

- The need for knowledge (how to . . .)
- The need for information (where can I find out . . .)
- The need for organization (who is responsible . . .)

- The need for direction (when and how should . . .)
- The need for development (prepare for the future . . .)
- The need for standards (what level of performance . . .)

Thus it is a high calling to become a supervisor. But with this high calling comes a challenge. Successfully responding to this challenge requires conscious and dedicated effort and the development of new skills.

CHARACTERISTICS OF EFFECTIVE SUPERVISION

Considerable research has been conducted to determine what traits are important in the area of supervision. Some of these factors can be best described in terms of personal characteristics or traits and others are best considered as issues of style. A few of the personal characteristics that contribute to the making of a good supervisor in the field of health care are as follows:

- *Solid foundation of technical knowledge.* Every supervisor must maintain a good base of knowledge and expertise. Not only is this expertise likely to be required in case of emergency, it is also necessary so that the supervisor can train new employees, develop regular employees, and evaluate the performance of the entire work group.
- *Ability to complete work through other people.* In today's society, this involves more than just being able to tell other people what to do. It means having the ability to exercise positive personal power and influence so the best possible results are achieved in the long-term.
- *Desire to achieve at high levels.* With current demands on organizations to perform at ever higher levels and with the increased scrutiny from every direction on the health field, underachievers simply will not be able to survive the rigors of supervision. If the personal desire is lacking, the group performance will be mediocre at best.
- *High expectations of achievement from others.* The pygmalion effect plays a strong role in the workings of management. As a strong supervisor once said, "If you think they will or if you think they won't, you're right." Maintaining positive expectations about the workers is one of the most valuable traits a supervisor can possess.
- *Confidence in one's own ability and the ability of the workers.* Because of the many pressures and challenges a supervisor will face, self-confidence is essential. But it is not enough. The supervisor must also be confident in the workers. Because of the nature of the role of the supervisor, this is not a separate issue. Since the supervisor is ultimately responsible for the performance of the workers, supervisory confidence also means worker confidence.
- *Ability to instill a sense of value in others.* For people to perform well, they must place a high value on the work they are doing. More than anyone else, the supervisor plays a key role in the shaping of these individual values on the job.

- *Ability to communicate.* Since the essence of supervision is completing work through other people, the ability to communicate is critical. But often when people think of communication skills in the context of supervision, they think only of sending skills. Listening skills are also important.

Even among those supervisors who possess these personal traits, there are almost as many styles as there are supervisors. Nevertheless, several elements of style that typify the approach used by many good supervisors include the following:

- Try to give general directions and instructions rather than focusing on specific details and constantly "checking to see if the workers are performing. To the greatest extent possible, develop the people so they can respond to direction that focuses more on the "what" than on the "how to."
- Clearly establish goals and objectives for the work group. People need to know exactly what they are supposed to accomplish.
- Invole the workers in many of the decisions. This is especially important for decisions that focus on the "how to."
- In general, avoid "crisis management"; instead, function at fairly low-key, low-pressure levels. Of course emergencies will arise, but the situations that require a supervisor to behave in a crisis-like mode should be few and far between.
- View the job of supervision in the context of helping the workers to be successful in their work. It is not advisable to act as though people need to be coerced or manipulated into doing a good job. Assume they want to do well, but will occasionally need help.
- Use worker mistakes as an opportunity to learn. Learning is an ongoing, lifelong process. On-the-job learning is facilitated primarily by the supervisor. The supervisor is primarily responsible for ensuring that mistakes do not happen more than once. As a supervising nurse once said, "The first time it happens, shame on the worker, but learn from the experience. The second time it happens, shame on the supervisor, because the proper training wasn't provided."
- Speak positively about the organization and the people who work in it. Good supervisors are not afraid to make a psychological commitment to their organization and its people. They also are not hesitant to stand up and be counted when it is the proper time to express this positive attitude.
- Stand up for workers when they have legitimate concerns to address or problems that need to be solved.
- Actively develop sound working relationships with the workers. The ranks of supervision are not appropriate places for a popularity contest. Nor is popularity a valid foundation for supervisor/subordinate relationships. But that does not mean a supervisor should ignore the importance of the relationship and fail to build an effective interface. The relationship should be established on mutual dignity and respect and should make it easy for the necessary information to flow in both directions.

- Assume both responsibility *and* authority for unit performance by taking the initiative to solve problems and improve performance. It also means confronting decisions that need to be made and acting decisively in the face of potential conflict.
- Freely give recognition and public praise to others in the organization, and especially to members of the supervisor's own work unit. In short, good supervisors do not compete for credit. They are quick to give credit where credit is due, while at the same time are modest in regard to their own contributions.
- Take the initiative to solve organizational problems. It is disheartening to hear a supervisor say, "Why doesn't management do something about this?" Or: "When will the administration solve that problem?" Supervisors *are* part of the management team or the administrative structure of their organization. The person who first notices a problem has the primary responsibility for confronting the problem and carrying through to see that it is solved. As a member of the management team, that is what he or she is paid to do. Passing the buck is not part of anyone's job description.

In essence, Supervisors must have a tremendous amount of role flexibility, because different kinds of demands are placed on them. How these different roles develop are discussed in the next section.

ROLE FLEXIBILITY FOR SUPERVISORS

An outline of the different needs that people have in regard to their supervisors was presented on page 7. To satisfy these various needs, a supervisor must be flexible in establishing different kinds of relationships in different situations.

In some situations, for example, the supervisor will be the *key person*. Workers, patients, or middle managers will turn to the supervisor for direction, information, knowledge, or help. In this role, the supervisor must be supportive and responsive. Technical expertise, problem-solving skill, and decision-making abilities will be essential for success. Confidence and decisiveness will often be the key traits that will determine success or failure.

Many times supervisors will be "caught in the middle" and will have to play the role of *mediator*. This situation often occurs when the workers see things differently from higher levels of management. It might also occur when two work groups develop opposing points of view. Or it could simply be a conflict or a personality clash between two individuals. All are examples wherein the supervisor will probably be asked to mediate the dispute and to solve the problem. These are cases in which communication and conflict management skills will be necessary for effective performance.

Because the first-line supervisor is still close to the work, however, a significant amount of time will be spent in the role of being *another worker*. In this role, technical knowledge and the wisdom that derives from experience are important.

Likewise is the ability to exercise positive peer leadership and the skills necessary to influence group dynamics as a co-worker.

Another situation that arises less frequently, but often places the supervisor in a sensitive predicament, occurs when upper management takes control to handle employees directly *without* involving the supervisor, thus leaving the supervisor in *a marginal relationship* with the workers. The most common example would be during labor negotiations. The management team negotiates directly with the union, and although the supervisor will be required to live with the outcome, little can be done to influence what the outcome will be. The supervisor must be careful to avoid "taking sides" or doing anything that might have an adverse effect on the results of the negotiations.

Frequently, people who work for the supervisor will develop problems. These may be personal problems, problems with other people, or problems that develop within the entire group. When problems such as these arise, the supervisor will have to become somewhat of a *human relations specialist* to be able to solve them. Counseling, consulting, and leadership skills will be important. In addition, the supervisor should also know something about group dynamics and organizational behavior.

SUMMARY

It should now be obvious why many people claim that the supervisory position in organizations is the most critical. In health care organizations, the job is particularly demanding because of the added responsibility for patient care. To the employees in the work group, the supervisor represents the organization. To the organization, the supervisor represents the primary contact point for the delivery of service. These two factors are not much different from the pressures felt by many supervisors. But the presence of patients complicates matters significantly. In some cases, the supervisor's decisions will literally mean the difference between life and death.

But with challenge also comes the opportunity for tremendous satisfaction and fulfillment. Few positions can provide the feelings of accomplishment and contribution that are typical of supervisory positions in health care organizations. The remainder of this book is designed to help supervisors meet the challenges and reap the rewards of one of the most fulfilling career choices available.

REFERENCES

Drucker, P. *Management: Tasks, Responsibilities and Practices*. New York: Harper & Row, 1974.

Management for Supervisors. A booklet prepared for Northern Natural Gas Company based on extensive review of research. Omaha, NE:, 1979.

Morrisey, G. L. *Management by Objectives and Results for Business and Industry* (2nd ed.). Reading, MA: Addison-Wesley, 1977.

Stoner, J. A. F. *Management*. Englewood Cliffs, NJ: Prentice-Hall, 1978.

PART TWO

THE FUNCTIONS OF HEALTH CARE SUPERVISION

Chapter Two

Planning

Planning is usually listed as the first function of management because here the activities of management begin. If the essence of supervision is to produce results through people, then planning is the logical first step, because it is through planning that one decides which results are to be produced. Without knowing which results one is attempting to achieve, it is useless to try to fulfill any of the other functions of management. In short, planning is the most basic of all supervisory and management activities.

Due to the nature of health care service delivery, planning may be one of the least natural activities for health care supervisors to implement. Most health care services are provided on a reactive basis—a patient becomes ill, and the health care provider reacts to the illness by diagnosing and then treating the illness. The decision about what to do is based on what else happens first. Thus everyone—physician, nurse, and allied health professional—when performing the technical or operating work in the health care field is conditioned to function in a reactive mode. The way most services are provided, however, little opportunity is afforded for people to take initiative or to be proactive.

However, planning is a proactive function. It requires taking initiative. Anticipatory thinking is the essence of all planning activities. As supervisors in health care organizations shift their focus from individual patient care to the organized delivery of health care on a broader scale, it is important they understand this distinction. Organizational needs are different from patient needs. Organizations cannot afford to wait until something happens to decide what to do about it. Such an approach to running an organization would guarantee failure. On the contrary, supervisors in organizations must anticipate needs and be prepared to meet them.

DEFINITION OF TERMS

One popular definition for planning describes it as the process of deciding what to do, when to do it, how to do it, and who is to do it (Steiner, 1969). In addition, several terms, which have special meaning in the context of management planning, are used to help define different levels of purpose within an organization. By understanding the meaning and relevance of these terms, one can also better understand the elements of planning and the activities that are included in the function of planning. The most common definitions of these terms include the following:

- *Superordinate goals*—the primary goals, which include philosophically oriented or value-based statements that give deep meaning and feeling to an organization's intent. These statements describe the "spiritual fabric" of an organization and convey the underlying values that top management cherishes. Good organizations will have clearly defined superordinate goals. Recent research has revealed them to be a common denominator for achieving excellence (Pascale & Athos, 1981).
- *Mission*—an organization's purpose or long-range reason for being. Every organization has its own unique purpose and reason for being. It is important to know the specifics of the organization's purpose and how all the activities in one's area of responsibility relate to it.

Contrasting missions can be seen, for example, in comparing an acute care facility to an extended care facility. The mission of the acute care facility would focus on providing a broad range, complicated, or perhaps unrelated services to a cross section of the community. On the other hand, the mission of the extended care facility might be to provide skilled nursing to the elderly. Both missions are important and identify a vitally needed purpose. But they are clearly different and describe a totally different context and type of operation for each.

- *Goals*—short- and long-range major accomplishments that lead to the fulfillment of the mission. The distinguishing characteristic of a goal is that it addresses a *major* accomplishment. For example, a goal for the acute care facility might be to add a new trauma center. A goal for the extended care facility might be to add a new wing to its current facility in order to increase the number of patients it might be able to serve.
- *Objectives*—statements of measurable results to achieve. Objectives are tangible and almost always measurable in some way. Objectives are also specific, containing explicit statements of results, dates for completion, and cost factors. An example of an objective might be: To complete the implementation of the new computerized accounting system by June 15 with contract costs not to exceed $68,000 and training and coordination costs not to exceed 400 work hours. Another example might be: To correct all discrepancies identified in the accreditation visit by September 30 at a cost not to exceed $1300 and 48 work hours.
- *Standards*—statements of results to be achieved on a continuing basis. Where objectives focus on single key results to be accomplished, standards focus on ongoing performance. An example might be: To process all routine lab work within one hour from the time the work is submitted. Also referred to as *Performance Standards* in many organizations.

- *Plans*—written documents that contain mission, goals, objectives, and the detailed supporting information necessary to accomplish the desired results, including staffing, budget, and scheduling information.
- *Schedules*—detailed listing of all the activities that must be carried out to achieve the desired results. Each activity is programmed with specific dates and time frames for completion. Schedules are included as part of the plan.
- *Budgets*—detailed listing of all the resources required to reach the objectives. Resources are usually divided into three categories. The first is human resources which we keep track of in terms of work hours, days, months, or years. They might also be accounted for in terms of labor costs, personnel overhead costs, or work-year equivalents.

The second category is materials and supplies. This category typically includes consumable items and working inventory and is usually accounted for in terms of dollar cost.

The third category includes facilities and equipment. This category typically includes real property, buildings, major equipment, and tools that are purchased for long-term use.

- *Staffing plans*—detailed listing of the personnel requirements for different operations and activities. Usually this listing describes requirements in terms of number needed, position descriptions, job titles, and professional titles rather than individual names.
- *Policies*—general guidelines for making decisions. They define the operating ground rules for the organization. Policy helps to channel individual thinking and behavior so these will be consistent with the mission, goals, and objectives of the organization.
- *Rules*—stated requirements for specific behaviors in different situations. Rules are more explicit than policies and, rather than serving as guides for decision making, they serve as substitutes for individual judgment. In other words, where the rules apply, there is usually no need for exercising judgment; one simply follows the rule as stated.
- *Standard operating procedures*—set of detailed instructions for carrying out a sequence of activities that occurs fairly frequently. Used to maintain consistency in operations and to reduce the likelihood of error. Also referred to as Standard Procedures (Morrisey, 1977; Stoner, 1978).

A final term that is commonplace in the world of management today is the term *Management by Objectives,* often referred to simply as *MBO.* The phrase was identified by Peter Drucker in the mid-1950s. Since that time, it has caused considerable controversy and some confusion for supervisors and managers.

At a recent session of the National Institute on Health Care Leadership, a medical director asked: "Do you think MBO is good or bad?" When asked what he meant by this question, the medical director explained how his hospital had tried to implement a management by objectives program and how badly it had failed. He cited numerous problems and described in great detail the many difficulties he encountered because of the new approach.

This medical director's experience is not unique. Similar outcomes have resulted in numerous organizations, both in and out of the health care field. But these failures do not make MBO good or bad. To blame the failure on the concept is inappropriate, to say the least.

Managing to accomplish objectives is the essence of all management and supervisory activities. Managers and supervisors have a simple primary role—to ensure that the results of the organization are accomplished. Objectives are merely statements of results to be achieved. Thus all managers and supervisors manage by objectives. However, some identify and state their objectives clearly, while others tend to be more vague.

The problem with some of the more formal MBO programs is that they become so formal and so highly structured that they become self-defeating. The procedure for identifying and communicating objectives can be so complex that people spend more time trying to satisfy the requirements of the system than they do in trying to perform the work. Supervisors then become the victims of the system rather than the beneficiaries.

Planning is not something one does for its own sake. Planning is only beneficial to the extent that it helps one to achieve one's intended results more efficiently. But it should also help one to be more effective in dealing with factors external to the organization and in identifying what results one should pursue. To this extent, it is an enabling activity, not a producing activity. Thus one should always strive to make certain that all planning activities are approached in the proper frame of mind.

Guidelines for effective planning and ways to manage by objectives in a simple, straightforward manner will be presented later in this chapter. But first it is important to understand the benefits of good planning.

BENEFITS OF GOOD PLANNING

Intuition alone has never been a completely reliable basis for making organizational decisions. This statement is particularly true in the complex field of health care. One reason is the field is so complex. Another is that the stakes are high—human lives are involved. Planning provides a rational framework for making decisions regarding the present and future operations of the organization. But this is not the only benefit to good planning. Several additional benefits are also worth noting, such as the following:

- *Good planning helps to minimize risk and uncertainty.* Through the use of more rational techniques for making decisions, planning helps to develop more logical approaches for handling major organizational issues. Planning provides a structured way to ensure that leaders in the organization keep up with current developments in technologic, social, and economic conditions that are constantly changing.

- *Good planning helps to ensure the best possible use of all resources.* Health care organizations achieve results through the effective use of personnel, facilities, supplies, equipment, money, and time. It is impossible to expect that all will be used to optimum benefit without deliberation and forethought.
- *Good planning helps to focus the attention of staff on achieving the organization's goals.* Not only does this make it easier to use and coordinate the organization's resources, it also makes it easier for individuals in the organization to know what is expected of them. In addition, it makes it easier for people to exercise their own judgments productively and to take initiative to contribute to the aims of the organization.
- *Good planning provides one with points of measurement for evaluating performance and measuring productivity.* Benchmarks, or points of reference, are important to ensure that the right results are being produced. They reduce the likelihood of wasted effort or erratic performance.
- *Good planning increases the likelihood that the organization will be effective—meaning that the organization will do the "right" things.* It is possible to be efficient but not effective. In other words, one can do what one does well, but be doing the wrong things.
- *Good planning helps the organization keep abreast of change.* From now until the twenty-first century, no other field will experience more change than the health care field. Many of these changes will occur at a more rapid rate than did those of the past. Consequently, experience and intuition will have less benefit, and planning will have greater value.

In addition to these overall benefits, a number of more specific benefits are achieved through good planning at the supervisory level. These include the following: (1) the accomplishment of work on schedule; (2) elimination of waste and reduction in other costs; (3) improvements in the quality of work; (4) better job control; (5) equipment and materials needs can be identified in a timely manner; and (6) workers can be assigned to work at their highest skill levels.

With all these benefits, why don't supervisors always plan? Or why don't they plan well?

BARRIERS TO GOOD PLANNING

Planning activities are impeded by two categories of factors. The first category is comprised of those factors that primarily focus on the supervisor alone. These factors include skill deficiencies, personal reluctance, and so forth. The second category includes factors that may be more organizational in nature. They include other factors such as a reluctance on the part of others to commit to planning processes or to the plans themselves; lack of adequate planning guidelines in the organization; or simply widespread poor management. A more detailed analysis of a few factors follows.

- *Lack of knowledge and skills.* Many supervisors in health care organizations simply do not know how to plan because the training has not been provided on either a formal or informal basis.
- *Lack of understanding of the organization and its subunits.* Because a thorough appreciation is lacking, many supervisors feel uncomfortable trying to influence what happens within the organization. They tend to be more reactive rather than pro-active and this dampens enthusiasm for planning.
- *Reactive posture of health care.* As mentioned earlier in the chapter, most health care services have typically been delivered in response to a problem. People in the field have thus become comfortable with responsive thought processes rather than anticipatory thought processes. This approach is exactly the opposite of what is needed to be successful in management.
- *Lack of understanding of the external environment.* Competitors, regulatory agencies, and the general public are all part of the external environment that must be handled effectively if an organization is to succeed. However, because supervisors do not completely understand these groups, they have a tendency to shy away from the planning activities that are essential for influencing them.
- *Inadequate support from others in the organization.* When planning is not an integrated practice throughout the organization, it is difficult for an individual supervisor to be effective in this area. Often, because budgets are tangible documents and concern the future, budgeting is confused with planning. In fact, in many organizations, the budget process is a substitute for good planning. Budget preparation is not planning. Acting as though it is means falling into a trap that will guarantee mediocrity.
- *People in the organization do not use plans properly.* Plans introduce change. People frequently resist change because they are comfortable doing the things they have always done and doing them the way they have always done them. Thus they become reluctant to use plans because to do so would mean moving away from an established comfort zone.
- *The planning approach used is wrong for the organization.* Although there are a number of guidelines worth following, there is no "one best way" to plan. Frequently, however, a manager will take a successful approach from one organization and attempt to force that approach onto another. Frequently, the results are frustration and failure.
- *Planning activities focus on the wrong amount of detail.* It is easy to err in the direction of either too much or too little detail. As a general rule, the higher a person is in the organization, the less he or she should be involved in details. When top management becomes too involved in detail, chaos results. The same happens when supervisors and workers overlook important details.
- *Plans are used to control rather than to inspire and lead.* Plans should not be used to coerce members of the organization, nor should they be the basis for blaming and finding fault with performance. To the contrary, they should be the guiding mechanisms that inspire people to perform and show them the direction to go.

These barriers to effective planning pertain to the correctness of application. None of these barriers pertains to the validity of the planning function. Planning is not only always appropriate, it is also essential. But if it is to achieve its purpose, a number of guidelines must be followed.

GUIDELINES FOR EFFECTIVE PLANNING

Several factors determine the overall effectiveness of planning. The following guidelines for improving planning practices will help you achieve optimum success (Lyles, 1982):

1. *Ensure proper input.* The supervisor should carefully ensure that all affected organizational units and individuals are involved appropriately in the planning process. This does *not* mean all must participate equally. Each will not have equal contributions to offer. But the supervisor should make every effort to ascertain that everyone who has something to contribute does so.

2. *Make plans specific and measurable.* General plans are meaningless. Vagueness causes confusion. The more specific a plan is, the better it will work.

3. *Be realistic.* There is a persistent myth among many managers and supervisors that it is wise to set goals that are too high to be achieved. They think, ''So what? Even if they don't achieve them, I will have gotten the best from my people.'' Not likely. People like to stretch, but they also like to succeed. If the goals are so unrealistic that everyone knows they cannot possibly be met, they will lose their enthusiasm from the outset.

4. *Avoid overplanning.* Resist the urge to become involved with excessive detail. Do not include a large number of unnecessary items and do not waste time writing about events that will happen anyway. The goal of planning is to make us better supervisors—not to make us better documentarians or historians.

5. *Do not underplan.* It is easy to develop plans that ignore the routine requirements that exist in all organizations. An example would be to schedule the operating room for one case right after another in such rapid succession that there is no time in-between for the routine cleaning and restocking that must be done. Do not become so driven by key results that sustaining results and routine performance suffer.

6. *Communicate the plan.* More good plans fail because they were inadequately communicated than for any other reason. After you plan your communication strategy, ensure that complete communication is effectively accomplished. To be properly carried out, plans must first be understood.

7. *Allow for contingencies.* Flexibility is a key to success. If one becomes too rigid, one becomes fragile and brittle. In the pursuit of our goals, new events will arise and they will bring with them new information. New information

necessitates new decisions. Make room in your plans for these decisions to be considered and the plans changed when necessary.

8. *Assign clear responsibilities.* Joint responsibility or dual responsibility is no responsibility. Clear definitions of both responsibility and authority give people the freedom to act in pursuit of your goals. Many frustrated supervisors have clear goals and unclear responsibilities and never realize the source of their frustration is the resulting confusion about who is supposed to do what.

9. *Troubleshoot plans prior to implementation.* The most cost-effective kind of problem solving a supervisor can perform is problem solving in advance. This method involves solving problems before they actually become problems and reach crisis potential. After planning, stand back and ask what can go wrong with the plan. Then correct any discrepancies that are discovered. (Lyles, 1982)

Follow these guidelines and it will be difficult to go astray in the challenging area of planning. But prior to covering the details of how to prepare a plan, one additional topic should be understood as background information. This topic is *forecasting*—in essence, how to take a realistic look at the future so that we know which issues our plans should address.

FORECASTING—HOW TO LOOK BEFORE YOU LEAP

Planning concerns the future. Unfortunately, no one has yet developed a method for predicting the future with any consistent degree of reliability. But there are methods for taking at least some of the guesswork out of future developments so that you can be as well prepared as possible to handle future challenges. These methods are included under the heading of forecasting.

Forecasting is the technique of assessing present conditions and trends to determine what the future will be like. It is done not to make the supervisor a fortune teller, but rather to enable the supervisor to take the steps that will most likely prepare for future events in the best manner possible. This is why forecasting is a necessary prelude to planning.

Analyzing present conditions and projecting them into the future cause the supervisor to anticipate demands that may be placed on the work group and identify potential problems and future needs for development. To do this adequately, the supervisor must assess equipment and material needs as well as the strengths and weaknesses of the work group. Today's assessment helps prepare for tomorrow's demands.

One reason many supervisors fail in forecasting is that they do not adequately understand their current situation. It is unlikely that a supervisor would be able to project the capabilities of the work group into the future if those capabilities are misunderstood.

Another reason supervisors often fail in forecasting is that they do not listen to the experienced people around them, including other supervisors and experienced managers. New supervisors in particular should find more expreienced supervisors to be a good source of counsel when assessing the future of operational demands.

The actual steps a supervisor should take to conduct a thorough process of forecasting prior to commencement of planning activities are quite straightforward. They include the following:

1. *Assess present capabilities.* A thorough review of employee capabilities, equipment, technology available, materials, and support services should be conducted.

2. *Review past performance requirements.* Make sure to understand fully the demands of the past. These should include both emphasis on the amount and level of production and the quality and type of service your group is expected to meet. Take note of both cyclical and constant requirements. Also try to identify emergency or nonroutine demands.

3. *Predict future demands.* As best as possible, using past experience and the opinions of experienced people, define the needs your group will be asked to meet in the future. Think in terms of quantity, type, and quality of production and service.

4. *Assess areas of potential weakness.* Identify the demands you might not be able to meet. Think through possible courses of action that might be followed to overcome these deficiencies.

5. *Review your forecast with others.* Ask qualified people to evaluate your work and explain the areas with which they agree and disagree. Be sure your immediate supervisor is one of those with whom a discussion takes place.

Once the forecast is completed and there is general agreement that it is the best that can be defined under the circumstances, it is then time to start planning. Now is the time to begin to make the decisions about how the future will be handled.

As we discuss the ''how to'' of planning in the following section, remember that our primary concern here is with supervisors. Strategic planning or top management planning will not be discussed in great detail. Rather, we will focus on the supervisor's role in planning and we will examine the steps that will be most beneficial to supervisors when they are fulfilling this role.

HOW A SUPERVISOR SHOULD PLAN

Planning should begin before you assume the responsibilities of supervision. This preliminary planning should focus primarily on the values, ideals, and standards that you will reflect as a supervisor. These will become the basis for the superordinate goals you will establish in your new role and which will give meaning and significance to your efforts and the work of the people in your group. What is the image you and your group will project?

At this stage of the process, you must avoid generalities and think about the specific nature of your work and its distinguishing characteristics. Will you emphasize service? If so, what exactly do you mean? Do you mean efficient service, like that found in a production line or cafeteria? Or do you mean humanistic, caring service like that found in an intensive care unit?

What comes first in your organization? The patient's feelings, wants, and needs? Or is the urgency and quality of care more important?

We can say all these are important all the time, but that does little in helping us to lead our work group. The balance of each will vary depending on the circumstances and the type of work involved. For example, in the emergency room, quick, correct, and efficient delivery of care might be of overriding importance. At the same time, in the recovery room, although monitoring and care are important, additional concerns such as patient comfort and wants may gain in importance.

To what extent should teamwork be stressed rather than individual performance? Precision versus speed? Which people represent the organization to outsiders? Who is responsible for keeping internal relationships working smoothly?

How will terms like professionalism and excellence be defined and explained to members of the work group? What do these things mean in the context of daily operations?

It will be important to be able to portray a vision of what is important and what will be emphasized as you assume your supervisory responsibilities. This is what determines whether people will take pride in working with you or will just consider their time spent with you as "time on the job." It is also the primary determinant of what outsiders will feel about you, the people who work with you, and the organization as a whole. Thus answering the following questions in specific detail will help develop the superordinate goals for your group:

1. What values will be most important for you in this position? Why?
2. What actions will you take and expect others to take that will demonstrate belief in these values?
3. In the context of the work this group is trying to accomplish, what traits describe professionalism?
4. What standards of excellence should be expected from the members of the group?

Initially, it is important to answer all these questions by yourself. After several months on the job, considerable benefit will be derived by having the members of the work group spend some time together reviewing them and refining them to add more detail and substance. Then, once a year, the group should revise them, adding more detail and ensuring that the necessary changes evolve over time. They should also be reviewed with new employees as part of their orientation program.

The remainder of the supervisor's planning activities can be divided into two areas of activity: operational planning and budgeting. A distinction is made here between the two concepts because they are often confused as one. Most often, budgeting is seen as a substitute for planning. Budgeting, however, follows operational planning, as will be explained later.

Operational Planning for Supervisors

The first step in operational planning is to define the unit's mission or long-range reason for being. Why does your work group exist? What key results is it expected to achieve? Why are you on the payroll? Why are the people in the work group on the payroll?

The mission statement describes your group's ongoing purpose. This statement of purpose breathes life into daily work activities and provides a sustaining sense of direction. It is the background against which individual goals are set and decisions are made. The mission also provides consistency and stability. Although the mission may change occasionally, it will normally undergo only slight evolutionary adaptations over time.

It is also important to describe how the mission of the work group ties into the mission of the total organization. This description helps you to remember the big picture and ensures that the activities of the total organization are coordinated.

Perhaps the best example of an organization that has survived and performed well over the years because of a clear definition of mission is the Red Cross. Since 1863, the mission of the Red Cross has been to prevent misery in time of war or peace and to serve all peoples, regardless of race, nationality, or religion. Many countries have failed to survive this long. Few organizations can boast of the same level of accomplishment or contribution as the Red Cross.

The key to the success of the Red Cross has been the clear understanding and dedication to this purpose. The organization has not diverted its energies with specific political goals nor has it shown favorites. The people who work in the organization and the outsiders who come in contact with it know and understand its focus. Thus there is little confusion about what to expect from the organization. Both insiders and outsiders share common expectations, making it easier for the organization to perform and make the contributions it does.

On a smaller scale, the same will be true for your work group if the mission is clearly defined. People will know what to expect and they will have a clear understanding of the focus of effort. They will also understand how their actions relate to the total organization.

Define the mission by answering the following questions:

1. What key results does your work group exist to produce?
2. What is your group's most significant contribution to the organization?
3. What is your group's most significant contribution outside the organization?
4. In one or two sentences, describe your group's purpose or long-range reason for being.

Your response to the last item will be the group's mission statement. After having spent the necessary time to think it through, test your definition with others in the organization to see if it also makes sense to them. Avoid giving this issue only cursory attention. Be willing to continue to modify your statement until it truly represents the essence of what your group is aiming for. Do not copy others. Your mission statement is the guiding light for your work group, it should be unique to you.

Next you should set goals. Goals are statements of short- and long-range major accomplishments that will contribute to the fulfillment of the mission. You will decide whether to set the goals on your own or jointly with other members of your work group. In either case, you will want to solicit input from the people in the group. They will have a number of good ideas about what can be improved in your operation. They will also have a keen sense of what needs are not being met adequately among the people whom you serve. These areas are the best for seeking out possible goals.

A good guideline is to have about four to six major goals that you are striving to achieve. Too many are likely to cause frustration because they will compete with the ongoing routine work assignments and regular duties each person must accomplish. Too few, however, will lead to lax work habits and boredom. The challenge of accomplishing something meaningful is important to people, so do not be afraid to set high goals and maintain high expectations so that people will want to achieve them.

To set goals, first review the results of your forecasting efforts and answer the following questions:

1. What future demands, challenges, or problems are likely to confront your work group?
2. What needs are being unmet or are likely to arise in the future?
3. What can we contribute to the organization to make it better for the people we serve?
4. What can we contribute to the organization to make it better for the people in it?
5. What can we do to increase efficiency?
6. What can we do to make the organization perform better?
7. What are the goals of higher management?
8. What are goals of other units in the organization that we are in a position to support?
9. What does higher management want us to do that we have not been doing?

From the answers to these questions, it should be possible to state quite a few meaningful goals. Be sure they are not too general. Although they should be major accomplishments, they should also be fairly specific.

After identifying goals, the next step is to set objectives. Like goals, objectives should also be tied to the goals and concerns of others in the organization, including higher management. Objectives are specific statements of measurable results to be achieved.

When people say they are managing by objectives or using management by objectives, all they are saying is that they regularly identify the results they want to achieve, state them in the form of objectives, communicate these intentions to others, and follow through until they are accomplished. The more clearly their objectives are stated, the better they are communicated; and the more rigorous the application, the better the person is managing.

The following guidelines will help you to set good objectives:

1. *Make sure objectives are clear.* Morrissey (1977) suggests the following format for writing objectives to ensure optimum clarity:

   - Write the word "To" followed by an action verb
   - Write a single key result to be achieved.
   - Write the word "by" and state the date by which the objective is to be achieved.
   - State the maximum cost to achieve the objective, in dollars and/or workhours.

   Thus the format would appear as follows:

   > To *[action verb] [single key result]* by *[date]* at *[cost not to exceed]*.

2. *Objectives should be challenging.* Nearly everyone likes a challenge, particularly if it is related to his or her professional and/or technical skills. Few workers have ever walked off the job solely because they were challenged in the area of work performance. This is especially true in the health field where people expect demanding performance and take pride in accomplishing worthwhile goals.

3. *Objectives should be reasonable and achievable.* Unreasonably high objectives hurt both morale and performance because they generate a sense of failure when they are not achieved. Objectives must be capable of being achieved in a reasonable time frame with a worthy amount of effort.

4. *Objectives should be measurable.* The only way to know if results are being achieved is to be able to see some tangible indicator. Progress and results must be quantitative to be meaningful. The measurement does not necessarily have to be numerical, however. It could just as easily be represented by a milestone or the production of a key output. But whatever the measurement, it should be specific and tangible to eliminate doubt concerning whether the desired result has been achieved.

5. *Specific time frames for achieving objectives should be set.* Deadlines help to prioritize work activities and also convey the appropriate level of urgency that should be associated with different objectives. Time frames help in coordination and also in allocation of different resources.

6. *Objectives should be used to manage.* Quite often, supervisors set objectives then set them aside until the following year when someone asks them to think about objectives again. This is poor management. Objectives should be used and reviewed on an ongoing basis to direct the efforts of the work group. They should be revised and updated as new objectives arise and as old objectives are achieved.

7. *Individual accountability should be assigned for each objective.* There is no such thing as dual accountability or joint accountability. To minimize confusion and ambiguity, each objective should be assigned to one particular person to achieve. Responsibility should thus be clear and everyone should know exactly what is expected of him or her and everyone else.

With these guidelines in mind, setting objectives should be a relatively simple process. The following procedure should suffice:

1. Review the results of your forecast.

2. Review the missions and goals of higher levels of the organization.

3. Review your own mission and goals and evaluate your performance against any previously set objectives.

4. List the primary results you would like to achieve during this upcoming performance period.

5. Obtain input from your subordinates about results they think are important for the future of your work group.

6. Either jointly with your subordinates, or by yourself, formulate a list of objectives that adhere to the format described in the above guidelines.

7. Review the objectives with your supervisor, amending as necessary.

8. Discuss the final list with your subordinates (either jointly, individually, or both) and assign individual responsibility and deadlines for achievement. Also establish dates for reporting interim progress toward the achievement of the goals.

After formulating objectives, you will often need to develop action plans, schedules, budgets, and staffing plans for the achievement of certain objectives. Not all objectives will require such detailed planning. However, certain lengthy or complicated projects or programs will benefit from such activity.

It is best to let the person responsible for achieving the objective decide the details of how it will be accomplished. This procedure allows the supervisor to stand back and be used as a resource rather than doing much of the work that can be accomplished better by others. It helps the supervisor avoid detailed work and make a better contribution to a wide variety of projects. But, perhaps most important, it gives the person doing the work more true responsibility and ownership of the project. Whenever a supervisor can focus primarily on the "what" and can avoid the "how to," he or she will be better off.

A simple format for outlining a plan of action is presented in Figure 2.1. Note that the goal is first stated clearly at the top. Then potential obstacles and resources are outlined in the following boxes. The project is then outlined in the remaining spaces, with dates in the left-hand column, activities to be carried out in the center, and specific results at each phase of the process listed on the right. There are several advantages to using a format like that in Figure 2.1. First, it eliminates confusion. The consistent use of a standard format will aid in understanding what is intended and in what sequence activities will be carried out.

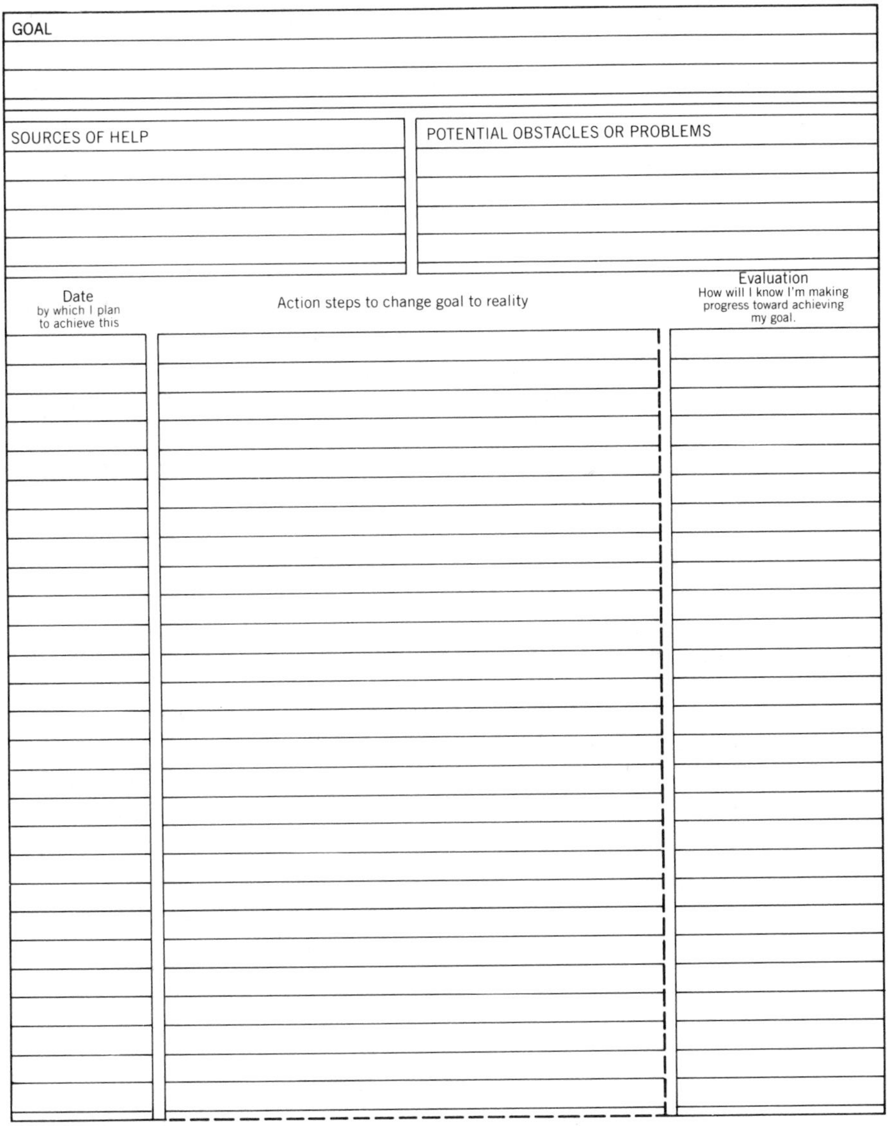

GOAL	

SOURCES OF HELP	POTENTIAL OBSTACLES OR PROBLEMS

| Date
by which I plan
to achieve this | Action steps to change goal to reality | Evaluation
How will I know I'm making
progress toward achieving
my goal. |
|---|---|---|
| | | |

Figure 2.1. A sample format for outlining a plan of action. (Courtesy of M. Wayne Wilson, San Diego, California.)

Another advantage is that it simplifies communication. When ideas are transmitted in a form that everyone is familiar with, they are easier to understand and respond to. Expectations can be clarified early to avoid confusion once the work has begun.

Rarely, if ever, will a supervisor be called on to carry out planning in more detail or in greater scope than is outlined above. *The key to success is in knowing how to define mission, set goals, define objectives, and outline an action plan that will achieve the objectives.* Master these skills and you will never be faulted in the planning function. As you apply these techniques, you will be surprised at how easy it will become to start new directions and breathe new life and energy into both your work group and the entire organization.

SUMMARY

Planning is the beginning function of management. Planning activities create the framework within which all other activities take place. Health care supervisors should be especially careful to ensure that proper planning occurs, since they may be reluctant to shift into the proactive mode that planning requires.

Good planning involves anticipating future events and preparing to deal with these events as they arise. But, most important, it means identifying the specific results your organization will attempt to produce and developing the strategies that will most likely produce them.

REFERENCES

Lyles, R. I. *Practical Management Problem Solving and Decision Making.* New York: Van Nostrand Reinhold, 1982.

Morrisey, G. L. *Management by Objectives and Results for Business and Industry* (2nd ed.). Reading, MA: Addison-Wesley, 1977.

Pascale, R. T., & Athos, A. G. *The Art of Japanese Management.* New York: Simon & Schuster, 1981.

Steiner, G. A. *Top Management Planning.* New York: Macmillan, 1969.

Stoner, J. A. F. *Management.* Englewood Cliffs, NJ: Prentice-Hall, 1978.

Chapter Three

Organizing
and Staffing

At the supervisory level in health care organizations, the functions of organizing and staffing interrelate. Although the supervisor's role in organizing is not as extensive as the role of middle management and higher administration, it is important. Most of the supervisor's organizing activity feeds directly into the staffing function. Thus these two functions are discussed and analyzed in this chapter.

The first part of the chapter presents the basic principles of organizing that a health care supervisor should know and understand, whereas the activities a supervisor will often perform are explained at the end of the section.

The second part of the chapter focuses on the staffing function. The health care supervisor's role in staffing is of prime importance. Nothing can be accomplished without good people being in the right place. Good staffing ensures the presence of good people, while good organizing ensures they are in the right place so that the goals of the organization can be accomplished.

ORGANIZING

The following is taken from James Stoner's book, *Management:*

> The need for sound organization is well illustrated in the *Old Testament, Exodus* 18:13–26. Following the exodus of the Israelites from Egypt, Moses found himself the sole judge of the disputes that arose among the people. Consequently, the people "stood by Moses from the morning unto the evening," waiting for him to make decisions. Jethro, the father-in-law of Moses, saw this spectacle and realized that little could be done with such an unwieldy organization. He offered his advice, thereby becoming the first recorded management consultant. If we translate the language of *Exodus* into modern management jargon, we find that Jethro's advice to Moses has a decidedly contemporary ring:
>
>> And thou shalt teach them ordinances and laws, and shalt show them the way wherein they must walk, and the work that they must do. [Establish policies

and standard practices, conduct job training, and prepare job descriptions.]
Moreover, thou shalt provide out of all the people able men . . . and place
such over them, to be rulers of thousands, and rulers of hundreds, rulers of
fifties, and rulers of tens. [Appoint men with supervisory ability and establish a
chain of command.] And let them judge the people at all seasons; and it shall
be, that every great matter they shall bring unto thee, but every small matter
they shall judge. [Delegate authority and work tasks and follow the *exception
principle*—that is, allow routine problems to be handled at lower levels and
settle only the big, exceptional problems yourself.]

The obvious effect of this proposed reorganization, which Moses adopted, was to
save Moses time and effort. This in itself is no small accomplishment; increased
efficiency is one of the desired benefits of the organizing process. However,
Jethro's suggestions in fact accomplished a great deal more; they permitted Moses
and the Israelites to achieve their goals. Moses' main aim was to lead his people
to the Promised Land; yet he was spending all his time settling disputes. The
Israelites' main aims were to carry out God's commandments and follow Moses;
yet they were spending all their time awaiting Moses' rulings. Through Jethro's
reorganization plan, Moses and the Israelites were freed to carry out their major
responsibilities. [For example, an Israelite who, after learning the law, still
needed a ruling could quickly obtain one from a supervisor and proceed with his
or her job.] As a result, the Israelites were able to move more rapidly toward the
Promised Land. (James A. F. Stoner, Management, © 1978, p. 222–223. Reprinted by permission of Prentice-Hall, Inc., Englewood Cliffs, New Jersey)

Organizing is the second function of management. Once the initial planning has
been completed, it is necessary to organize the available resources so the necessary
activities can be performed to accomplish the organization's goals. In planning, we
identify the desired results to be achieved. In organizing, we identify the activities
that must be performed to achieve these results and then we provide the structure
that will best enable accomplishment. The term *structure* includes policies, standard
operating procedures, work rules, and information systems, as well as job descriptions and organizational charts.

DEFINITION OF TERMS

Organizing means to create the most effective grouping of activities (allocation of
work) together with the necessary guidelines and coordinating systems so that the
organization's goals can be achieved as efficiently as possible. Organizing is not an
end in itself. But good organizing is more than merely a means to an end. It is a
prerequisite for good performance. Without good organization, the people doing the
work will not be able to perform. Although good organization will not guarantee
good performance, if good organization is lacking, performance will suffer (Drucker, 1974).

If carried out properly, organizing will provide clear identification of (1) responsibility, (2) authority to make decisions, (3) functional separation of work activity,

and (4) expected levels of performance for individuals and groups. A universally perfect organizational structure does not exist. Every aspect of management, including organizing, is situational. What will work best for one organizational will not necessarily work best for another. In organization, the best goal to strive for is simplicity. The more simple the structure, the better. The more complicated the structure, the more that is likely to go wrong—the more problems supervisors will have to solve that are caused by the organization itself. Fewer problems are caused in simply designed organizations than in complex ones.

Several terms relating to the function of organizing that should be remembered include the following:

- *Division of work*—identification of the discrete tasks and individual work activities that must be performed. This analysis occurs at the beginning of any organizing activity so the building blocks of the organization can be identified; often referred to as *task differentiation.*
- *Coordination of work*—arranging the tasks and work activities in the most logical flow so the work itself can be performed in the most efficient manner possible. This is often accomplished by examining the decisions that are required, the information that must be exchanged, or the relationships between different types of work; often referred to as *task integration.*
- *Organizational chart*—a diagram of the functions and positions in the organization, showing how they relate to one another. Levels of responsibility and functional groupings are also conveyed.
- *Formal organization*—the organization and relationships that are officially derived by the organizational chart. The formal organization describes the way the organization is supposed to work.
- *Informal organization*—working relationships within the organization that are outside the boundaries of the formal organization or are inconsistent with it. The informal organization is how the organization actually does work that is at times different from the way it is supposed to work.
- *Position description*—a written statement of the content, responsibilities, and authority of a specific job. In the past, many organizations made a distinction between job descriptions and position descriptions. Position descriptions were used to describe jobs at the managerial level and job descriptions were used at the operational level. Today, however, most organizations use the term position description for both.
- *Span of control*—the number of subordinates who report directly to a supervisor, less often referred to as *span of management.*

Structure always follows strategy. Thus the work of organizing should always follow the work of planning. First we decide what to do; then we decide the best way to allocate resources and organize our activities to attain our goal. For example, consider the differences between a small community clinic and a large acute care hospital.

The small community clinic adopts as its primary purpose the mission of providing routine health care to the surrounding community. It is likely to be run by one or two physicians who hire a small staff of nursing and allied health professionals. The physicians themselves may do much of the administrative or management work when not providing health care or they may hire a group practice manager to handle these duties. Either way, most of the organizing efforts will be handled informally and most of the relationships and interactions will occur on an informal basis.

On the other hand, the large acute care hospital will have numerous departments, each with a large number of physicians with different specialties, and a large administrative staff. Each department will be run with a large degree of autonomy. Coordination of effort between departments will be on a fairly formal basis and considerable attention will be paid to rules, policies, written guidelines, and structured communication processes. People in positions of responsibility will be required to spend a higher percentage of their time making the organization work and a lower percentage directly providing services. The larger and more complicated an organization becomes, the more of everyone's time is required to make it work efficiently and effectively.

However, regardless of the size of the organization, care should be taken to ensure that it is organized properly and that it is designed to run as efficiently as possible. Time spent in organizing activities will pay positive dividends in the long run.

BENEFITS OF GOOD ORGANIZATION

The primary benefit of good organization is that it provides the structure that allows the institution to achieve its goals and fulfill its mission. This benefit alone should be sufficient justification for organizing activities. Nevertheless, several additional benefits can also be gained from good organizing, such as the following (Stoner, 1978):

- *Good organizing provides for greater efficiency.* Whereas planning provides for greater effectiveness (that is, doing the right things), organizing provides for greater efficiency (doing things right).
- *Good organizing frees people to act.* Once people know what their responsibilities are and have clearly defined boundaries of authority, they will possess the freedom to take initiative within those boundaries. They should not feel as though they will be punished for taking initiative.
- *Good organizing clarifies expectations regarding performance.* Once responsibility and authority are clearly defined, people should have a clear sense of what they need to do to satisfy the requirements of their position and to fulfill the needs of the organization.
- *Good organizing eliminates duplication of effort.* If activities are properly coordinated, there should be no wasteful duplication of effort. Not only is the wasteful duplication avoided, but people should be able to do each discrete activity better, knowing everything that will be achieved by everyone else.

- *Good organizing reduces the amount of conflict.* Conflict often rises in organizations because those involved are confused about their individual roles and responsibilities. Clarifying individual roles and responsibilities facilitates good organizing, which thus reduces most causes of conflict on the job.
- *Good organizing instills confidence.* Eliminating much of the doubt and confusion about job responsibilities facilitates good organizing, which thus helps people gain confidence that their individual efforts are contributing to the success of the total effort.
- *Good organizing frees people to concentrate on their major tasks.* By thinking through certain organizing issues once and then following those guidelines, people will spend less time working through the same issues over and over again each time new activities arise.

These benefits make a compelling case for effective organizing in any organization. But before discussing the details of how it is done, we will examine some of the barriers that typically impede effective organizing practices.

FACTORS THAT HINDER GOOD ORGANIZING

Most of the factors that impede good organizing practices result from one of two things. Either they are related to knowledge or skill deficiencies on the part of the people who should do the organizing, or they result from bad attitudes regarding the benefits of organizing. The primary factors include the following:

1. *Empire building.* Many times organizational productivity is seriously undermined through overstaffing. It is important that health care supervisors keep their work groups in the proper perspective, maintaining a balance of functions and capabilities that are consistent with overall objectives and needs. Empire building should be discouraged by ensuring that the relative importance of any position is not determined by the number of people supervised. Importance should be based on a function's value to the organization and its contribution to overall goals (Rantfl, 1978).
2. *Myths about structure.* A few supervisors and administrators in the health care field believe that people do not like structure. The myth is that people suffer adverse effects in morale and motivation when they work in a structured environment. The reality is that all people perform better when the organizational structure is clear and appropriate to the objectives of the organization. Thus good structure facilitates effective performance; it does not detract from it.
3. *People lack Training in the technology of organizational design.* Some organizations are designed improperly simply because people do not know how to design them correctly. Organizational design is a skill like any other management skill. Understanding concepts such as span of control and coordination of work are essential to building effective organizational structures.

4. *Title inflation.* Organizational titles should be based on organizational needs. They should not be used as rewards or substitutes for money. Title inflation often leads to top-heavy organizations, increased overhead costs, and reduced organizational flexibility. Titles have value only when (a) there are relatively few of them; (b) they are awarded with consistency; and (c) they clearly stand on the merits of the positions and the individuals involved (Rantfl, 1978).

5. *Operational direction not defined.* Structure follows purpose. The organization cannot be designed to receive results effectively if those results are not specified. Thus planning is the first function of management that sets the direction for organizational activities. Organizational design is the second function of management, which builds the structure to accomplish those results.

6. *Structure too vague.* Organizational designers may feel as though they are providing themselves with flexibility and freedom by making assignments or writing position descriptions that are too general, unclear, or lack specificity. This practice leads to confusion, not constructive guidance. To achieve the guidance that is necessary from proper organizational structure and design, the design elements must be specified clearly. In essence, supervisory responsibility and decision-making authority must be defined in each level in the organization.

7. *Unnecessary functions.* Adjunct functions not only create a direct drag on productivity but they are also demotivating to people who are conscientiously trying to contribute. Unnecessary functions should be ruthlessly removed from organizational charts and from organizational activity (Rantfl, 1978).

8. *Too much organization—too many levels.* It is just as easy to overorganize as it is to underorganize. Too many layers cause redundancy in effort and misuse the time of people who must receive an organizational response to carry out their work. The best organization is the simplest. Furthermore, an organization with fewer levels is better than an organization with too many. Keep the size of the organization and its complexities to a minimum.

With these pitfalls in mind, let us examine some of the factors that should be considered when building an effective organization.

FACTORS TO CONSIDER WHEN ORGANIZING

A health care organization structure should represent the most effective grouping of functions to achieve the organization's objective. The structure should be a catalyst that aids in job completion. It should never be an end in itself but should be viewed merely as a means for achieving the best possible use of available resources. Organizational structures should clarify both responsibility and authority. It should clearly define where the buck stops and who can make which decisions. Organizational structure should also aid information flow. Channels for communication and responsibilities for seeing that information is transferred properly should be clearly defined.

To design an organization that is both efficient and effective, span of control should be assessed. Specific decisions should be made regarding the optimum span of control in different areas. The span may be broad or narrow depending on the nature of the organization, the work that is involved, and the type of people who will be carrying out the work. For example, in a high-risk setting, such as intensive care, span of control will tend to be narrow so that close supervision can be maintained. In a more general clerical function, span of control may be broad because the risks are not as high and the work is not as critical. Care should always be taken to avoid any trend toward top heaviness. A tendency often exists in organizations to add layers and layers of supervision and administration using span of control as the primary justification. This practice is particularly prevalent in health care where patient needs or patient care requirements can always be used as a compelling argument to add more supervision or to add additional layers of administration.

Needless activity should be eliminated. Old needs may become obsolete much quicker than people realize. This is particularly true in the health care field of today. It is a sad fact of life but new technology is replacing the need for some human activity. Many times people cling to old habits and traditional ways of doing the job because of emotional attachment with that particular approach. While we do not want to implement change solely for the sake of change itself, we must be sensitive to the times when change does foster improvements in organizational function. We must confront the emotional ownership of some of these old habits and let them go.

Another important factor to consider when organizing is that of overlapping functions and joint responsibility. Joint or dual responsibility is no responsibility. Overlapping functions should be avoided as much as possible. Dual or joint responsibility should be eliminated completely. The aim of the supervisor is to ensure that redundancy is kept to a minimum (Rantfl, 1978).

Although we often think of planning as being the only future-oriented supervisory activity, it is important that we keep the future in mind when we design the organization as well. Although we design an organization to meet today's needs, it is important that we realize the future is not far away. Transitions into future operational demands can be considerably facilitated by an organization's structure that was developed with those future demands in mind.

Although nothing positive evolves naturally in organizations, it is important for the health care supervisor to ensure that the organization's structure evolves with the demands of the organization. Organizing is an ongoing, evolutionary process. What is appropriate for today may be completely wrong for tomorrow. The organization that is designed to facilitate the work that current demands require is likely to be obsolete in only a few short years. Because the health care field is changing, its organizations must change with it to keep pace (Drucker, 1974).

Finally, keep it simple. There is no substitute for simplicity. But be specific; simple does not mean vague. Communicate the structure in a straightforward and concise manner that formally transmits the intent of the organization to those who will be required to work within its boundaries.

HOW TO ORGANIZE

First, determine what activities need to be performed. This step is usually called either *task differentiation* or *division of work activity*. List all the activities that need to be performed by members of a specific work group. What does the organization require and what functions are necessary to accomplish the goals and objectives that have been defined for the group?

Second, group these activities together in clusters that allow for ease and accomplishment. This step is usually called either *task integration* or *coordination of work activity*. These clusters then become the basis for position descriptions. In other words, at this step the supervisor is asking how the work can best be coordinated and how the different tasks can be combined to facilitate their accomplishment with the greatest amount of ease and the minimum amount of supervision.

Third, actually define specific positions on a position description form. Figures 3.1 and 3.2 contain the actual position descriptions that a California acute care hospital uses for a staff nurse position and a charge nurse position.

As can be seen from the two examples, a considerable amount of work is required to write the kind of position description that is required. The descriptions include a definition of the position, qualifications required, supervisory authority exercised, supervision received, physical requirements, safety responsibilities, work hours, committees and meetings the incumbent will be required to attend, promotional opportunities, and detailed listings of duties and responsibilities. It should also be noted that people from facilities other than this one might find these particular position descriptions inadequate for their needs. Positional requirements will vary from organization to organization. It is essential to analyze thoroughly the needs of your organization to specify the exact demands your organization requires.

After the position descriptions have been written, the actual structure of the organization is created. At this step, span of control becomes a consideration and the organizational chart is designed. The final step is to write necessary policies, regulations, and standard operating procedures and protocol. No structure is complete without these foundations to guide its activities. Policies should specify safety standards, decision-making protocol, and so forth.

When the correct organizational structure is in place, the next step is to bring the right people in to make it work. A big challenge exists today for the health care supervisor in the area of staffing. With the principles of organizing in mind then, let us move into that area. Once the structure is in place, we must breathe life into it.

STAFFING

The most important resources in an organization are its human resources. People who are willing to give their drive, talents, and energies make health care organizations work. The philosopher Plato is credited with stating that no two things can be held together without a third. No bricks can be held together without mortar. Words can be held together without glue, nails, or some other third element to bond them.

DEFINITION:

A staff nurse is a current California registered nurse who, under the direction of a Supervisor, Head Nurse has the responsibility for coordinating and evaluating the actual nursing care for an assigned number of patients, to perform a variety of professional nursing duties either in a general or specialized unit, and to function within the framework of the Nurse Practice Act. She/he is a professional consultant to the physician, responsible for the planning and implementation of nursing services specific for each patient under her care.

QUALIFICATIONS:

1. Graduation from an accredited school of nursing.
2. Possession of a valid and current license as a registered nurse, issued by the state of California.
3. Meets the health requirements of the hospital.
4. Can function under and meets standards of the Nurse Practice Act.
5. Knowledge of terminology, theory, techniques and practices of professional nursing, including the normal conditions of specialty to which assigned.
6. Knowledge of medicines and narcotics, along with their effects, side actions and contraindications.
7. Knowledge of a variety of specialized equipment.
8. Ability to develop and carry out a nursing plan.
9. Knowledge of the levels of nursing care expected (Nursing Process) and criteria used to evaluate nursing outcomes.
10. Ability to analyze facts and conditions and apply sound nursing principles in making decisions.
11. Ability to lead and assist in supervising the work of subordinate personnel.
12. Ability to communicate orally and in writing.
13. Ability to establish effective working relationships with physicians, patients, and fellow workers.
14. Demonstrated ability to accept and implement change.
15. Ability to implement the Total Nursing Process.

SUPERVISED BY:

Head Nurse/Shift Supervisor

SUPERVISES:

Other R.N.s, L.V.N.s, and/or N.A.s and W.S.s as directed.

PHYSICAL REQUIREMENTS:

Sitting, lifting, standing, bending in clinical units.

COMMITTEES AND MEETINGS:

1. Monthly unit meetings
2. All other meetings as requested

Figure 3.1. Job description: Staff nurse

SAFETY:

Responsible for maintaining and enforcing safety standards established for patient, visitors, and employees.

GENERAL DUTIES AND RESPONSIBILITIES:

1. Develop and carry out patient care plans and evaluate outcomes.
    a. Develop and update plan of care with patient.
    b. Formulate and implement discharge planning.
    c. Provide structured and informal teaching to patient.
    d. Initiate interdisciplinary referrals and patient conferences.
    e. Reinforce teaching done by other disciplines.
2. Demonstrate current knowledge of principles, techniques, and procedures of professional nursing.
3. Demonstrate current knowledge and practice of medication administration, and observe patients for response to prescribed medication and treatments, notifying physician when indicated.
4. Demonstrate knowledge and ability to operate equipment.
5. Perform procedures according to policy and procedure manuals.
6. Plan and organize work so that it is accomplished by the end of the shift.
7. Use time in patient area to maximum potential.
8. Use problem-solving techniques in decision making.
9. Recognize responsibility for own actions.
10. Report anticipated problems to physician or Head Nurse/Supervisor.
11. Identify questionable assignment and/or procedure and seek guidance.
12. Identify and intervene in crisis situations.
13. Identify and provide nursing intervention for patient needs specific to diagnosis.
14. Evaluate and update plan of care for expected outcomes.
15. Use problem-oriented approach and problem list.
16. Demonstrate complete and concise documentation.
17. Document specific observations relating to diagnosis.
18. Provide direct bedside care for daily routine and to carry out special treatments and/or procedures.
19. Observe and evaluate patient's signs, symptoms, and reactions to therapy in an effort to identify or interpret significant findings or changes that may require attention or notification of attending physician.
20. Demonstrate knowledge and practice of health in job performance.
21. Receive report from previous shift and give report to next shift.
22. Recognize limitations and seek guidance.
23. Initiate own research for self-education and staff development.
24. Assist physicians with treatments, dressing, tests, etc.
25. Give prescribed treatments and medications, adjusting to patient's condition.
26. Questions any order that may be unclear or that in the nurse's opinion could be detrimental to the patient's health.
27. Attends annual CPR review.
28. May be part of the Code Blue Team.
29. Assists in Title 22 and JCAH Standards enforcement.

Figure 3.1. (continued).

30. Maintain control of narcotics and medications.
31. Instruct patients or relatives concerning home care, in accordance with physician's instructions.
32. Initiate appropriate emergency measures that require independent judgment and action in order to sustain life.
33. Maintain or supervise maintenance of pertinent records.
34. Prepare equipment for treatments.
35. Assist in evaluating unit service and equipment.
36. Assist Head Nurse in the maintenance of clean, orderly, calm patient and nursing unit; also ensure proper temperature and humidity control and application of safety and environmental standards.
37. Contribute to and share in unit conferences, committee meetings, staff development and in-service training programs, and other procedures developed to improve service to the patient.
38. Participate in fire, safety, and disaster drills.
39. Practice infection control principles.
40. Promote a courteous atmosphere, demonstrating diplomacy with personal interaction.
41. Use established channel of communications.
42. Maintain knowledge and skills by attending in-service programs and continuing education seminars and workshops. Keeps informed of changes in nursing standards.
43. Is aware and understands the social, religious, cultural, and economic needs of patients and makes appropriate referrals.
44. Assists with inventory of supplies and equipment on unit.
45. Observes and reports any malfunctions of equipment on the unit.
46. Any other duties that may be assigned.
47. Assists in clinical orientation of new employees.
48. Assists in eliminating unnecessary waste.
49. Recommends changes in nursing policies and procedures to improve general nursing functions.
50. Assists in maintaining nursing standards of care.
51. Participates in research projects related to nursing.
52. Works with other departments in attaining and maintaining continuity of patient care.
53. Holds in confidence matters that are considered privileged information.
54. Is aware of other health organizations and their function in the community.

Figure 3.1.   (continued).

Can organizational resources—material, money, and time—be brought together to serve productive purposes without people? No—people make things happen.

However, we cannot rely on just anyone to accomplish the job. For the purposes of the organization to be achieved, the right people with the right skills and the right traits must be in the right place at the right time. It is the health care supervisor's primary responsibility to see that this situation occurs. This is the essence of the function we call staffing. Let us examine the function of staffing in more detail.

DEFINITION:

A registered nurse who is a proficient total care nurse, who demonstrates leadership ability to function as the resource person on the unit responsible for 8-hour management.

QUALIFICATIONS:

1. Graduate of an accredited school of nursing.
2. Currently licensed in the State of California as an R.N.
3. Flexible mature person who uses good judgment, logical priorities, and deductive reasoning in his/her nursing care.
4. Sufficient physical and mental health to meet job demands.
5. Shows a knowledge of basic anatomy and physiology, and is able to determine normal from abnormal.
6. Must be a skilled observer.
7. Demonstrates leadership abilities.
8. Functions within the Nurse Practice Act.

SUPERVISED BY:

Head Nurse of the unit.

SUPERVISES:

All nursing personnel of his/her shift.

PHYSICAL REQUIREMENTS:

Lifting, bending, standing, sitting, turning in patient care area.

SAFETY:

Responsible for maintaining and enforcing safety standards established by the hospital for patients, visitors, and employees.

HOURS:

2:45 P.M.–11:30 P.M.; 10:45 P.M.–7:30 A.M.; or as agreed by Director of Nursing.

COMMITTEES AND MEETINGS:

1. Attends monthly unit meetings
2. Other meetings as requested by Director of Nursing

PROMOTION TO:

Head Nurse if position is available and applicant is qualified.

Figure 3.2. Job description: Charge nurse

DUTIES AND RESPONSIBILITIES:

1. Same as Primary Care Nurse, see job description.
2. Demonstrates leadership abilities.
3. Makes out team assignments by acuity and instructs nursing personnel in their assigned duties.
4. Is aware of the assignment and load of personnel and assists them as needed.
5. Helps Total Care Nurse, if necessary, to assess needs of patient and priorities of care.
6. Assist in evaluating personnel on the unit.
7. Keeps Head Nurse informed of activities on unit.
8. Assists in improving staff skills and attitudes.
9. Assists in the orientation process of new personnel.
10. Helps total care nurses coordinate activities between patient and physician and other interdisciplinary departments.
11. Serves as the resource person on unit.
12. Understands and practices appropriate professional ethical conduct.
13. Participates in community workshops when possible.
14. Keep informed of changes in nursing and nursing standards.
15. Enforces hospital and nursing policies and procedures.
16. Works in cooperation with other departments in attaining and maintaining continuity of care.
17. Follows proper lines of authority.
18. Maintains good physical and emotional health, is well groomed, and uses good personal hygiene.
19. Holds in confidence matters that are considered privileged information.
20. Interprets philosophy, functions, and goals of nursing and the hospital patients, visitors, and community.
21. Assumes patient care assignment.
22. Other duties as delegated.

Figure 3.2. (continued).

What Is Staffing?

Staffing is the managerial function that ensures the organization will have sufficient quantity and quality of personnel to achieve its mission and goals. This is an ongoing challenge because of the constantly changing nature of the health care work force. Workers leave the organization through voluntary resignation, death, retirement, dismissal, and layoffs. People move about within the organization because of promotions, transfers, or demotions. As a result, supervisors must engage in staffing activities on an ongoing basis. In larger organizations, the demand is greater and more insistent. In smaller organizations, there is usually less mobility in the work force so the need to engage in staffing activities will be less and more sporadic. The following activities comprise the staffing function.

Human Resource Planning.   This planning begins with a thorough analysis of need for skills and staffing demands for the foreseeable future. Human resource planning is divided into short- and long-range demands of the future. Expected changes in the organization, including expansions, reductions, change in service mix, and level of patient care, are all factors that should be included in the needs analysis. As a result of the analysis, plans are developed for carrying out the other steps in the staffing process.

Recruitment.   Recruitment is normally carried out in collaboration with the personnel department. This phase of activity is designed to ensure that a qualified applicant pool exists from which supervisors in the organization can hire qualified personnel. This practice consists of communicating with the personnel department and outside sources about the employment opportunities that would exist or are likely to exist in the future. Activities usually involved in recruitment include advertising, visiting schools or colleges where graduates may be found, contacting state employment agencies, and personnel agencies, and working through present employees.

Selection and Hiring.   The selection process involves evaluating individual applicants from the applicant pool and selecting those that are most qualified for the various openings that arise. The hiring process consists of making offers to the appropriate selectees and bringing them into the organization. During the selection and hiring process, the supervisor will rely on application forms, resumes, interviews, references provided by the applicant, and perhaps examinations to determine competence.

Orientation.   This area is one of the most critical and most often overlooked activities in the staffing area. The objective is to ensure that the new employee enters and makes a smooth transition into the organization. Many critical attitudes, values, and expectations are established during the orientation phase of an employee's relationship with an employer. Accordingly, it should be managed carefully and efficiently by the supervisor.

Training and Development.   No one is brought into the organization operating at his or her full potential for the new position. For a person's full potential to be realized he or she must learn, grow, and develop that potential on the job for the particular position. The health care supervisor is responsible for ensuring that the training and development process is managed to ensure optimum growth and the best possible productivity.

Transfer, Promotion, and Demotion.   Transfer is a change in job assignments from one position in the organization to another. A promotion is a change that involves an increase in responsibility, with a concomitant increase in salary and/or status. A demotion is a shift to a position of lower responsibility, staff, or salary in the organization. Health care supervisors will be involved in managing all of these from one time to another.

Separation. This phase is often considered the final staffing function because it involves the termination of an employee's relationship with the organization. Separation is a function as important as any of the others. Separation may involve resignation, layoff, discharge, or retirement. The type and quality of separations and organizational experiences can give valuable insights into the organization's effectiveness. Poorly managed organizations typically experience a higher rate of separation. The more effectively managed organizations typically experience less separation and therefore less turnover. Good staffing practices also benefit organizations by preventing problems. Few things are more frustrating for a supervisor than confronting problems that arise from having the wrong people in the organization at the wrong time. The guidelines presented in each of the following sections will help prevent this kind of problem from arising (Stoner, 1978).

How to Conduct Human Resource Planning

Resource planning is the activity that ensures that the personnel needs of the organization are consistently met. This planning is achieved by analyzing current and anticipated skill needs, vacancies, and operational demands in the foreseeable future. After this analysis is completed, plans are developed for carrying out the other steps in the staffing process. For supervisors, human resource planning usually extends from six months to two years into the future. The following steps comprise the planning process.

1. *Analyze current staffing levels and demands.* This goal is carried out by first conducting an audit of currently allocated positions. Each position should be evaluated to ascertain that it is needed and relevant to the operations of its work group. After this existing staffing structure is thoroughly analyzed, further analysis should be conducted to gain insights into the dynamics of the structure in operation. How much overtime is required to meet operational demands? Is the amount of required overtime consistent with company needs and good supervisory practices? What are current turnover rates? In other words, are personnel changes within the group consistent with good supervisory practice? If problems exist in any of these areas, plans must be made to solve them so that routine staffing demands can be defined. A determination should be made regarding what ongoing staffing requirements can be expected on a regular basis.

2. *Assess future changes that will affect staffing demands.* Are there any anticipated changes in the volume or type of work the group will be asked to perform? Is the organization planning to expand? Will additional services be added in the near future? Are any reductions anticipated? What impact will these changes have on staffing needs? How much lead time will be allowed to have the right staffing structure in place when the changes occur?

3. *List the steps that must be taken to ensure future staff needs are met.* Plans for executing the other steps in the staffing process should be written. These steps should include recruitment, selection, cross-training, development, and layoff activities. Specific dates for accomplishing each step should be listed.

As soon as the plan is developed, activities should commence to see that it is carried out. Methods for carrying out the individual activities are detailed in the following sections.

HOW TO RECRUIT

The primary purpose of recruiting is to provide a pool of candidates large enough to enable the organization to select qualified employees as it needs them. In large organizations such as a major acute care hospital, the supervisor's role in recruiting will be minimal. For the most part, it will be the supervisor's responsibility to communicate anticipated staffing needs in a timely and explicit manner to the Personnel Department. It will then be the Personnel Department's responsibility to ensure that a qualified applicant pool is available to the supervisor. In smaller organizations, such as a modest-sized group practice, it may be necessary for the supervisor to carry out all the recruiting activities. In either case, it is useful for the health care supervisor to understand the issues and the activities involved with the recruitment process. The following procedures should be followed in recruiting.

1. *Review your organization's policies.* Many large organizations have a policy of recruiting or promoting from within the organization. In other organizations, seniority lists may be used to determine who will be selected to fill certain positions. Policies will require that vacancy notices be posted within the organization or within a specific department prior to recruiting outside that organization. Whatever policies exist in your organization, it is important that you understand them in detail prior to developing a recruitment strategy. Everything must be done within the boundaries of existing policy.
2. *List relevant sources for candidates.* Recruitment practices can suffer if the supervisor fails to consider all sources for obtaining candidates. A particular source for obtaining applicants will vary with different occupations and geographical areas. Some good sources include the following:

   - Employer's or trade associations
   - Public employment services
   - Private employment agencies
   - Direct hiring
   - Friends and relatives
   - Advertising in newspapers
   - Professional associations or journals
   - Colleges and universities
   - High Schools
   - Vocational colleges
   - In-house transfers
   - Transfers from other organizations

The supervisor is responsible for assessing these sources in accordance with organizational policy and existing hiring demands to determine which ones will be best for a particular situation.

3. *Determine optimum mode of communication.* The supervisor must find the best way to notify the various sources that a hiring need exists. Will a telephone call suffice? Should an explanatory letter with position descriptions enclosed be sent? Perhaps for some sources, personal visits by the supervisor to explain the need in detail may be the most appropriate way to communicate.

4. *Communicate the need.* Establish contact with the appropriate people for each candidate source. Ensure that true understanding of your hiring needs is conveyed and ascertain that cooperation will be forthcoming. Communication in this regard is not a one-time affair. Communication and coordination with various sources should be continuous and ongoing so that an adequate applicant pool can be maintained.

5. *Evaluate the response and adjust as needed.* Provide feedback to the various contacts in the applicant sources to ensure that the appropriate level of referral is maintained. Too few applicants in the pool at any particular time limits the supervisor's flexibility and might detract from being able to hire the most qualified people. On the other hand, having too many people in the applicant pool is likely to discourage potential applicants because word may spread that it is not worthwhile to apply for a job at that particular organization (Wilson, 1982).

Usually, when people say they cannot find qualified employees, they are making a statement about themselves and their own inefficient recruiting practices. Supervisors who maintain effective recruiting practices are rarely heard to complain of the shortage of qualified personnel. Each health care supervisor must ensure that a qualified applicant pool is in place at all times. From this qualified applicant pool, candidates are selected and hired to fulfill the needs of the organization.

HOW TO SELECT AND HIRE

Since capable people are the key to achieving your supervisory goals, substantial time and energy should be devoted to the selection and hiring process. Taking shortcuts here almost always causes problems later on that could have been avoided. A practical process for health care supervisors to follow in selecting and hiring new employees consists of the following steps:

1. Initial screening
2. Preliminary interview
3. Testing if necessary

4. Detailed interview

5. Final clearances

The steps are designed so that the least amount of the supervisor's energy can be expended at each step of the process to weed out the unqualified applicants. This practice will naturally allow for the most amount of time to be spent on the most qualified applicants to ensure that the best qualified are hired. Each step consists of the following activities (Dale, 1973).

Initial Screening

Initial screening consists of a review of all written information that exists for each applicant in the applicant pool. The supervisor should read through the files to examine application forms, resumes, letter of recommendations, notes from previous contact or records of previous contact with the applicant, and any other information that might exist regarding this applicant's qualifications or potential to contribute to the organization. At this step in the process, the supervisor should pay particular attention to past positions the applicant has held, the nature of prior responsibilities, salaries, length of time in each job, reasons for leaving, and the kinds of organizations the person has worked for. The goal of this initial screening is to identify a group of applicants whose qualifications and experience fit with the particular needs of the current opening. All applicants who appear likely candidates should be considered for the next step of the process.

Preliminary Interview

The preliminary interview may be conducted in person or via the telephone. A primary purpose for the preliminary interview is to determine if the applicant is still interested in the position. Quite frequently, applicant's needs or goals change after having filled out an application form, prior to being considered for a position by the organization. If the applicant has accepted another position two or three weeks prior to the opening becoming available in your organization, it is unlikely they will be interested in being considered for this opening. If the applicant expresses an interest in the position, the preliminary interview then provides the supervisor with an opportunity to gain early impressions concerning the applicant's interpersonal skills, motivation, attitudes, and other job-related qualities. A small percentage of applicants will invariably be screened out of the process at this stage. Those remaining in contention will be asked to proceed to the next step of the process.

Testing if Necessary

The testing step will not always be included as part of the selection process. Usually when it is included, the tests will be standardized tests or will be tests that have been developed specifically by the personnel department in a large organization. Testing is a particularly sensitive issue because of the laws pertaining to equal employment opportunity. Quite frequently in the past, when certain individuals have filed discrimination complaints relating to the selection process, they have charged that the tests used in the process of selecting applicants were discriminatory. It is almost impossible to prove that a particular test is not discriminatory, so it is risky for an individual supervisor to use a test that has not been widely accepted.

As a general rule, the criteria for a valid test in the selection process is that the test be job-related. The items on the test must specifically pertain to bona fide job qualifications. It is not only wrong but it is illegal to use tests that do not measure job-related qualifications. Thus general knowledge tests should not be used unless a requirement for the general knowledge contained in the test is a bona fide part of the job responsibility. As a general rule, for health care supervisors the best advice is to avoid administering tests. When tests are used, however, the supervisor should allow the testing process to be managed by the personnel department.

Detailed Interview

The detailed interview is perhaps the most important step in the selection and hiring process. It is in this process that the applicant's qualifications and potential are explored in as much detail as possible. The results of the detailed interview are used as the basis for making a hiring decision. Therefore, it is important that the interview be conducted as carefully and as deliberately as possible. The following guidelines should be followed to ensure this careful approach is carried out (Lyles, 1975; Rantfl, 1978; Steinmetz, 1971).

1. *Know the job thoroughly.* Use the position description, discussed earlier in this chapter, to conduct a detailed analysis of the requirements of the job. Ensure that, as a supervisor, all aspects of the job are clearly in mind before conducting the interview. Do not overlook any segment of the job because of unfamiliarity with the detailed requirements specified in the position description.

2. *Plan the interview beforehand.* Write down important questions that need to be answered. Ask general questions early in the interview and specific questions to fill in the gaps later. Use an interview format that has the questions written on a page with blank space to take notes and record the applicant's responses.

3. *Learn about each applicant before the interview.* Study the application and resume carefully. Pay particular attention to prior experience, training, employment patterns, and references. Identify specific areas of interest for each applicant so that unique strengths or weaknesses may be explored in detail.

4. *Maintain a comfortable atmosphere.* Allow sufficient time for the interview. Do not rush. Put the applicant at ease. Be friendly. Establish a relaxed, informal atmosphere. Be cordial. Encourage openness and free discussion.

5. *Provide information to the applicant about the organization.* Briefly describe the organization and the position for which the applicant is applying.

Explain any unique needs that might exist, but do not dominate the conversation. As a general rule, the applicant should talk 75 percent of the time.

6. *Use different kinds of questions.* Avoid asking too many questions that can be answered with a simple "Yes" or "No." Ask open-ended questions that encourage the applicant to talk about his or her abilities, experience, and accomplishments; then sit back and listen with your full attention. Also ask direct questions that provide the applicant an opportunity to provide specific information regarding his or her background.

7. *Encourage self-appraisal.* This process can often be achieved by asking hypothetical questions: "What would you do in a situation like this?" "In dealing with the following situation, what would be your strong points?" Opposing questions can aid in self-appraisal as well, such as: "What was your most challenging and least challenging past assignment?"

8. *Ask why the applicant wants to work for you.* How does this career change fit in with the applicant's overall career goals? What are the applicant's reasons for leaving his or her current position?

9. *Listen carefully.* Look at the applicant. Avoid reading the employment questionnaire or the resume during the interview. Do not shuffle paper while the applicant is talking.

10. *Give the applicant an opportunity to ask questions.* Many times the kinds of questions the applicant asks provide as much insight into the applicant's priorities and values as will his or her answers to the interviewer's questions. Remember the interview at this stage should be a two-way street. The applicant has concerns and needs as well and this is the time when those needs should be addressed.

11. *Close the interview tactfully.* Do not prolong the interview if the applicant is unqualified. Try to leave the applicant with the feeling that you are completely fair and objective. Let the applicant know when to expect to hear from you and what the next steps in the process might be.

Although the procedures for conducting job interviews are fairly straightforward, actually carrying them out effectively can be a formidable challenge. Many potential pitfalls exist along the way. When conducting the job interview, do not argue or criticize the applicant. It is unwise to register disapproval in the presence of the applicant for anything the applicant has said or done. Do not fall into the trap of trying to impress the applicant with your own importance. Moreover, you should not talk down to the applicant or interrupt the applicant when she or he is speaking. It is also unwise to try to anticipate the answers. Maintain an open mind at all times so that the applicant's responses can affect your decision about the person's capabilities. It is also unwise to try to trap the applicant or to create a stressful situation for the job interview. Although stress interviews were once considered by some to be beneficial, they are widely regarded as being inefficient today.

After all interviews are conducted, the data collected during the interviews are evaluated to determine which applicant will receive the job offer. At this step, however, the hiring decision is still a tentative one. It remains tentative until final clearances are obtained.

Final Clearances

In recent years, the number of people willing to falsify information on application forms and resumes has increased. Because of the critical nature of the health care field, the health care supervisor cannot allow the possibility that an employee may be joining the organization under false pretenses. After an applicant has been selected, therefore, the supervisor must contact references, previous employers, educational institutions, and other information sources to verify the information that the employee has represented in the application process. Some sources will be willing to provide more information than others. But all sources should be willing to verify basic information such as dates of employment, position held during employment, dates of graduation, and training received. The supervisor should also ask if the previous employer is aware of any problems in the applicant's work history. Occasionally, problems will be revealed, but more often than not the response to this question will be nebulous. Larger health care organizations have standard reference form letters that are sent out to references and educational sources to verify the information by mail. If there is sufficient time for written correspondence and verification of information, this approach can be useful. More often than not, however, the health care supervisor will be required to obtain such clearances via the telephone and use written notes as a record of the information that was obtained.

Many health care organizations also require physical examinations as a prerequisite for employment. If such examinations are required by your organization, it will be necessary to schedule them and to allow time for the results to be processed prior to clearing the employee for work.

After the supervisor has guided the applicant through all five steps of the selection process, the applicant is then ready to join the organization. The hiring decision is communicated to the applicant. It is important, however, that the new employee be brought into the organization as smoothly and as efficiently as possible. Thus another area of concern is orienting a new employee and bringing that person into the organization.

HOW TO ORIENT A NEW EMPLOYEE

An effective new employee orientation program begins each employee reports to work and extends through the first year of employment. The best way to examine the different elements of such a program is to analyze them in the context of the time frames in which they occur. The phases of an effective orientation program are as follows (Wilson, 1982):

Preemployment. Prior to reporting for work, the new employee should receive information from the organization concerning the following:

- The orientation program itself
- Employee benefits
- Dress code
- Parking, car pools, and transportation
- Where and to whom to report on the first day
- Information necessary for completing initial employee information forms

In addition, if the employee is relocating from a different geographical area, information should be provided concerning:

- Temporary living and transportation arrangements
- Real estate market and lodging conditions
- Relocation aids such as maps and community geography
- Information regarding schools
- Chamber of Commerce information packets

At this time, the employee's immediate supervisor should also ascertain that the organization possesses the employee's full name, starting date, telephone number, and other pertinent information. The information for the preemployment phase should be mailed to the employee in advance and should be followed up with a telephone contact to ensure the employee received the information and to welcome him or her to the organization.

First Day of Employment.   On the first day of employment, the supervisor should ensure that the new employee has adequate time to spend with the personnel department to allow the following to occur:

- Employee should complete all necessary organizational paperwork.
- Employee should review all company policies and specifically should become acquainted with policies regarding hours of work, dress code, pay periods, vacation days, holidays, sick leave policy, and other routine organizational policies.
- Employee should be provided with identification card or keys, parking permits, and other items necessary to gain access to the premises.
- Employee should receive an employee handbook or brochure describing pertinent organizational information of interest to the new employee.
- Employee should also receive written material outlining benefit plans and compensation plans in which the employee will be participating.

The first day of the new job can be stressful. The supervisor should do everything possible to make this time both relaxing and informative for the new employee. Specific time should be set aside to sit down in a quiet area and talk about the work group, the organization, and the policies and regulations that will affect the employee immediately. A tour of the department and all associated work stations should be made with careful attention to introductions that are businesslike, respectful of all parties, and friendly. During the introductions, the supervisor should make a positive association between the new employee and the work the group is doing. Anything that will reduce the curiosity of current work group members toward the new employee will be helpful. The tour should be scheduled in a logical format so that after it is completed the new employee will better understand how his or her job relates to the total organization's operations. This gives meaning to the work. The attitude and sincerity of the supervisor at this time is as important as anything that will be said. The relationship that is established at this time will have a tremendous impact on subsequent interactions between supervisor and employee. Many organizations use video tapes today as part of their first day orientation to acquaint new employees with the operations of the organization, including the magnitude and scope of what the organization is involved in. It is also an important time to outline the chain of command. It is important that the employee knows whom to report to in the absence of the supervisor or when problems arise and the supervisor is not present. How much time is spent with the employee during the next week or two will depend on the employee, the job, and the operational demands that exist. It is important to realize, however, that it is almost impossible to spend too much time with a new employee during these first days on the job.

Two Weeks after Starting.   A meeting should be scheduled with the new employee after that person has been on the job for about two weeks. Although the meeting should be formally scheduled, the discussion during the meeting should be informal. The purpose of the meeting is to determine if the employee has any misunderstandings or is unclear about any of the following areas:

- Work group practices
- Department operations
- Organizational history
- Reporting relationships
- Personnel policies
- Individual job responsibilities
- Work relationships with co-workers
- Any other concerns the new employee may have

Many times, concerns in these areas arise but are never adequately addressed by the supervisor. This can be one of the most critical sessions in the orientation program even though it is seemingly unstructured.

Thirty Days after Commencing Employment.   A meeting should be scheduled between employee and supervisor. The purpose of this meeting is to focus more specifically on the employee's performance and development in the new job. Although employee concerns in areas such as personnel policies, reporting relationships, and so forth can be discussed if need be, the primary focus of this meeting should be on performance counseling. How well is the employee adjusting to the work assignments he or she has been given? Is the job clearly understood and is performance at an acceptable level?

Ninety Days after Commencing Employment. Approximately three months after starting, the employee should again meet with the supervisor to discuss performance. Once again, employee misunderstandings or concern about other information areas should be considered, but the primary focus of the meeting should be on the employee's performance and development. Specific feedback should be given to the employee and expectations for continued performance should be outlined. By this time, the employee should have a clear understanding of the performance standards against which he or she will be evaluated. A comparison of current performance to those standards should be made and clearly communicated to the employee during this meeting. If there are problems regarding the employee's performance, appropriate problem-solving activities should take place. Written documentation of the employee's performance during this 90-day period should be completed by the supervisor and shared with the employee.

Six Months and One Year after Commencing Employment. At approximately six months and again at approximately the end of the first year of employment, another performance meeting should be conducted between supervisor and employee. In both cases, documentation of the employee's performance, using standard performance appraisal forms, should be completed by the supervisor and shared with the employee. At the 12-month meeting, the supervisor should also expand the conversation to include discussion about the employee's long-term career plans and how they correspond with the organization. It is important that the issue of career plans be opened with the employee prior to the end of a full year's employment with the organization. From this point forward, the employee should be treated not as a new employee but as a standard employee with goals and objectives that are unique but important to the organization.

It is impossible to underestimate the impact of an effective new employee orientation program on new employees. Virtually every study that has been conducted in this area in recent times has shown that it is one of the most critical activities that a supervisor can carry out. It is during this orientation period that the foundation is established for the new employee's relationship with the organization. If it is built well, the relationship will be a good one. If it is hastily thrown together, the prognosis is more dismal.

How to Train and Develop Employees

Developing employees is an ongoing process. It is the supervisor's responsibility to ensure that this process is consistent and viable. In today's operating environment, it is unreasonable to assume that the formal education an employee possesses when hired will carry him or her through the term of employment. It is even more unreasonable to assume that the formal education acquired at the beginning of one's career will sustain a person throughout the career. In terms of practicality and usefulness, informal, on-the-job training has often proved superior to formal education. Although a combination of both formal and informal education on an ongoing basis seems most desirable, it is the supervisor's primary responsibility to ensure that the informal education and training on the job is provided adequately.

A number of strategies for achieving effective on-the-job training have been devised. Among the most common that a health care supervisor will use include the following:

- *On-the-job training and problem solving.* The supervisor is responsible for using problems that arise in the course of normal operations as learning opportunities. This is the primary mechanism by which we learn from experience. Every experience should be viewed as an opportunity for enhancing development.
- *Special projects.* Assigning employees different projects that carry with them diverse responsibilities and challenges will stimulate the development of individual capability. A person does not have to know everything about a specific assignment before it is made. When people are given work to do, most often they will learn what they need to know to be able to accomplish the work on time.
- *Job rotation.* Rotating people through different positions or expanding assignments in a specific position will help develop a person so that he or she is capable of being assigned higher levels of responsibility and growth.
- *In-service training.* Organization-sponsored training programs can be tremendously helpful in the acquisition of specialized knowledge. Most large organizations sponsor in-service programs on a regular basis. Smaller organizations must rely on programs sponsored for the public, in local colleges, or by professional associations.

The health care supervisor must realize that, regardless of the educational approach taken, the greatest benefits accrue when employees are motivated to take the initiative and to accept personal responsibility for expanding their own work-related knowledge. In training and development on the job, the supervisor's emphasis should always be on self-development rather than on forced training. Several other factors can also help determine the effectiveness of organizational training. The most effective training occurs when supervisors accept the responsibility for training and do not rely on the training department or on the in-service director to provide such opportunities.

Furthermore, it is the quality not the quantity of training that is important. Learning can be even more valuable if it occurs on the job under the supervisor's competent direction than if it occurs in isolation under hypothetical classroom circumstances.

When selecting people to provide training, it is important to choose the best performers. It is the successful performers who consistently conduct the best in-service training. The volunteers who merely want to teach turn out to be the weakest trainers. Weak trainers inevitably cause poor learning to occur.

Training and development involve more than merely transferring information. The ultimate test for effectiveness is whether the trainees are motivated to apply the knowledge and skills presented. Application will never be achieved if the supervisor is unwilling to set the appropriate example and to instill in the subordinates a desire to achieve the highest standards of performance possible.

SUMMARY

Organizing and staffing are closely interrelated at the supervisory level in health care organizations. Both are enabling functions that allow the work activities and the performance of the organization to be carried out at the highest possible levels. They provide the framework within which directing and controlling activities can be conducted. Both organizing and staffing require sensitivity, insight, and understanding on the part of the supervisor. It is these activities that will determine whether the supervisor has the right people in the right place at the right time to be abe to achieve the results he or she is being paid to produce.

REFERENCES

Dale, E. *Management: Theory and Practice.* New York: McGraw-Hill, 1973.

Drucker, P. F. *Management: Tasks, Responsibilities, Practices.* New York: Harper & Row, 1974.

Lyles, R. I., & Wilson, M. W. *Practical Management Guidelines.* Self-published booklet, 1975.

Rantfl, R. M., et al. *R & D Productivity.* Culver City, CA.: Hughes Aircraft Company, 1978.

Steinmetz, L. L. *Interviewing Skills for Supervisory Personnel.* Reading, MA: Addison-Wesley, 1971.

Stoner, J. A. F. *Management.* Englewood Cliffs, NJ: Prentice-Hall, 1978.

Wilson, M. W. *Staffing: An Internal Development Paper.* Houston: The El Paso Company, 1982.

Wilson, M. W., et al. *Effective New Employee Orientation Programs.* Houston: El Paso Company, 1982.

Chapter Four

Leading

The topic of leadership is receiving considerable attention these days. Best sellers such as *In Search of Excellence, The One Minute Manager, Megatrends, Theory Z,* and *On People Management* all point to the benefits of having and using an effective style of leadership.

In some sense, leadership is probably the most important of the management functions, because the fundamental requirement of a manager is to ensure performance of employees. Since leadership can be defined as the act of "influencing others' behavior toward desired ends," we can see that performance results in part from an effective leadership style.

DEFINITIONS OF TERMS

Managers have long been interested in identifying leaders and promoting them to positions where they can impact performance positively. Despite the interest, however, leadership remains a rather nebulous topic. It is hard to train someone and guarantee that the person will become an effective leader. One reason for this difficulty is that leadership involves "style", and "style" is hard to teach.

There are numerous definitions of leadership. The one we prefer to use is as follows:

Leadership is the act of positively influencing employee behavior toward the achievement of personal and organizational goals.

Other terms that we will use in this chapter are as follows:

- *First-line supervisor*—the level of management in the organizational hierarchy that supervises nonmanagers solely.
- *Linking pin*—a term to describe the relationship in which a manager or supervisor "links" the organization above to the individuals below a particular manager or supervisor.

- *Reward power.*—the use of rewards to influence behavior.
- *Coercive power*—the use of threats or force to influence behavior.
- *Legitimate power*—the organizationally sanctioned power that derives from the management position occupied.
- *Referent power*—power that derives from the charimsatic appeal or personality of the leader.
- *Expert power*—power derived from possessing an expert knowledge base in a particular area.
- *Trait approach*—an approach to leadership that tries to identify physical, social, emotional, intellectual, and other characteristics of effective leaders.
- *Behavior approach*—an approach to leadership that assesses the way leaders act or the style leaders use in different situations.
- *Situational leadership*—an approach to leadership that is based on a style that depends on various factors.
- *Universal leadership*—an approach to leadership that specifies the one best way to lead.
- *Managerial grid*—a leadership model that describes the leader's "concern for production" and "concern for people" in a two-dimensional model.

BENEFITS OF EFFECTIVE LEADERSHIP

Although the benefits of having and using the appropriate leadership style should be rather evident, we will highlight some of the more important ones.

- Effective leadership influences behaviors and, in turn, leads to performance. Since performance is of interest, leadership is also of interest.
- Employees' morale and satisfaction states are higher if an appropriate leadership style is used.
- Managerial promotions and other rewards are based on the success of the leader.
- The role of the leader is far more satisfying and rewarding when the correct leadership style is used.
- The organization as a whole is stronger and performance will be higher when appropriate leadership styles are used by its leaders.
- The other parts of the management process, such as planning, organizing, and controlling, are more easily undertaken if the leadership climate is a positive and proper one.

THE ROLE OF THE SUPERVISOR IN LEADERSHIP

It can certainly be stated that all managers are supervisors and, therefore, the terms can be used synonymously. In a more narrow perspective, the term supervision refers to the first level of management in the organizational hierarchy. Accordingly, supervisors direct the activities and manage the work of nonmanagers. This role is a unique one because all other managers supervise the work of other managers. In this section, we will emphasize some of the leadership issues raised by the uniqueness of the supervisor's role (Robbins, 1984).

In addition to the fact that supervisors supervise nonmanagerial people, several other characteristics also make the leadership role of the supervisor unique. According to Robbins (1984), supervisors are required to do the following:

• Rely on technical expertise
• Communicate "above and below"
• Handle conflict created by the role of supervisor
• Handle added responsibility while having their authority restricted somewhat
• Be the representative of management to the employees

Supervisors must understand the jobs they supervise. A large proportion of the supervisor's time is spent handling the technical aspects of a particular job. Requirements and requests similar to the following are often brought to the supervisor:

• What to do if a machine breaks down?
• What to do if spare parts and raw materials run low?
• What to do about bottlenecks in production processes?

Since the employees in the supervisor's unit are performing nonmanagerial tasks, the items that would be brought to the supervisor by these employees would also be nonmanagerial and, in fact, technical in nature. This requirement to be technically proficient in addition to being managerially proficient is more pronounced for the first-line supervisor than for any other level of management.

Rensis Likert referred to the supervisory role as a "linking pin" concept (Likert, 1961). In other words, the supervisor links those organizational units above to those units or employees below. In the case of the first-line supervisor, the people above are managers and the people below are nonmanagers. The needs, drives, ambitions, and educational backgrounds of the two groups are often different and the supervisor will be required to use different communications styles, strategies, and procedures.

The role conflict derives from the in-between position of the supervisor. Supervisors are managers in one sense but are often not accepted as real managers. Since the supervisor may still wear a uniform, punch a time clock, or get "dirty" on the job. Furthermore, higher level managers often have college degrees and enter the organization from the outside, while supervisors are often promoted from a non-managerial employee status to that of supervisor. Furthermore, if promoted from within, supervisors have to leave old friends and sometimes these factors cause role conflicts.

The last unique characteristic of the supervisory leadership role is that, in the eyes of many employees, the supervisor is THE organization. Since rules, procedures, and policies are implemented by the supervisor, the employee sees the supervisor as THE representative of the organization. The phenomenon is even more exaggerated for shift workers who may rarely see a management representative except for the supervisor.

Since the supervisor is the last link between the organization and the employee, the role is an important one. If the nonmanagerial employees are the people who actually produce the produce or service of the particular organization, the supervisor is in a key position to influence positively or negatively through a particular leadership style that output.

THE ELEMENT OF POWER IN LEADERSHIP

Since power has been called ''America's last dirty word'' (Schermerhorn, 1984), we want to focus on power as an essential component of the leadership equation. We will describe the bases from which leaders derive their power and conditions that limit the use of a particular base. ''Power is an essential leadership resource'' (Schermerhorn, 1984, p. 308). We earlier defined leadership as the act of influencing behavior toward desired ends. Managers use power as the facilitating mechanism through which leadership is exercised. Although the word *power* is sometimes associated with negative issues, such as abuse, coercion, or dictatorship, it can also be a positive term because managers and supervisors have to use their power to accomplish the job through others. Power becomes a means to an end, and not the end itself (Albanese & Van Fleet, 1983).

The bases from which managers derive their power are the following (French & Raven, 1962):

- Reward power
- Coercive power
- Legitimate power
- Referent power
- Expert power

Reward power refers to factors such as pay, praise, promotions, and recognition that managers and supervisors use to influence behavior. The basic premise is expressed in the following communication: ''I have some rewards. If you will cooperate and do what I ask, I will give you some of them.''

Coercive power refers to processes such as censure, threats, demotion, firing, and assignment of unpleasant tasks that are used to punish people if they do not cooperate. This reward base is used in the following way: ''If you don't do what I ask, you will be sorry. Therefore, you had better cooperate and perform as I request.''

The third basis of power is referred to as a legitimate one. This power base is derived from the official, organizationally sanctioned power and authority that a leader has because of the role occupied. For example, a director of nursing has power because the organizational chart, job description, and other formal mechanisms provide it.

These first three power bases are associated with the position that the leader holds. The organization provides the leader with the capacity to reward, coerce, or administer legitimate power. The last two power bases are from a personal base in contrast to the organizational ones above.

Referent power derives from charisma or magnetism possessed by effective leaders. It has nothing to do with the first three bases of rewards, coercion, and legitimate power, but instead exists within the person. People are willing to allow their behavior to be influenced (our definition of leadership) merely because the leader has some personality feature or personal characteristic to which they can refer or with which they can identify.

The last power base, expert power, is also personal in nature and stems from the situation where the led are willing to cooperate because they believe that the leader has more knowledge about a particular situation than they do.

Effective leaders are (1) aware of the multiple sources of power, (2) know when to use a given source, and (3) work to strengthen those areas where the power base may be weak at a particular point.

Enhancement of the rewards power base is derived from following the "different strokes for different folks" message. People value different rewards and the supervisor should provide the desired rewards if the power base is to be expanded.

Most managers and supervisors do not like to use punishment but there are occasions when it is the appropriate way to influence behavior. Anderson says, "Discipline should be used consistently, should be tied directly to the poor performance, and should be administered in a nondefensive, problem-solving way" (Anderson, 1984).

Legitimate power is used more effectively in the following ways (Anderson, 1984):

• A problem-oriented position is taken.
• The supervisor ensures that the problem is understood.
• Confidence and decisiveness prevail.
• Follow-up procedures are implemented.

To develop a stronger referent power base, the following suggestions are made (Anderson, 1984):

• Show a strong interest in employees.
• Treat everyone fairly.
• Be a strong spokesperson for the group when communicating with higher management.
• Spend a considerable amount of time at the workplace.

In developing the expert power base, the manager should explain "why" when providing expert information rather than just flaunting the more extended knowledge base.

Even though there are multiple power bases from which managers can draw, we have all seen situations in which managers are not able to influence behavior in the preferred way. In other words, something limited the manager's influencing ability. Barnard provided a major foundation for understanding this limit by describing authority from an "acceptance" perspective (Barnard, 1980). A manager can have power, issue a number of directives, and make requests, but the power is realized only when the person "accepts" the request. When a supervisor makes a request or issues a command, one of two things occur (Schermerhorn, 1984). If the person accepts the request on command and performs as intended, the supervisor has power. On the other hand, if the person to whom the request or command is directed does not respond, the supervisor does not have power. The employee's degree of acceptance establishes the limits of supervisory power. Barnard (1980) stated that orders and requests are more likely to be accepted when the following conditions are met:

- The employee understands fully the action or behavior that is being requested.
- The employee believes that the necessary skills and abilities are possessed.
- The employee believes that the request is in the best interest of the organization.
- The request is consistent with the employee's personal value set.

The harder the supervisor works on behavioral, communication and leadership skills, the greater should be the acceptance proportion of the total requests made. Remember that until the employee accepts the request or directive, the leader does not have power.

Albanese and Van Fleet (1983) summarize the perspective that supervisors and managers should have regarding power:

Managers must use power. They must feel comfortable with it and seek to enhance their power base and sources. Power is a necessity of organizational life and the managerial styles. The necessity of power should not be negatively construed. Personalized power is negative, concerned with personal aggrandizement and power over others. Socialized power is positive, based on congruence between the interests of self and others and power through others. The essential role of power is as a means, not as an end. In reality, power is often sought for its own sake and for the satisfaction its possession brings. It cannot be denied that power is sometimes viewed as a second-level outcome to which individuals attach a very high positive valence. In such cases, an increase in power per se serves as a strong positive reinforcer. While there is nothing wrong with this view of power, from a managerial and organizational perspective, power is a means of achieving personal and organizational ends. For managers, power is a means of pursuing their own self-interests, but it is necessarily more than that. It is a means by which managers serve the interests of others, and, through that service, enhance their own interests. (p. 208)

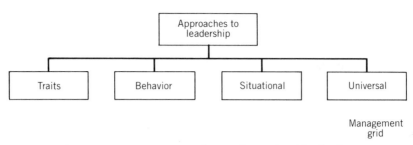

Figure 4.1. Major approaches to the study of leadership.

APPROACHES TO THE STUDY OF LEADERSHIP

"Although leadership is one of the most widely studied concepts since management, there is substantial disagreement as to what leadership is and how a person
should act as an effective leader" (Schoen & Durand, 1979, p. 17). With this reality
before us, we will review four different approaches to leadership as depicted in
Figure 4.1 (Flippo & Munsinger, 1982). This four-part breakdown of leadership
represents essentially all the approaches that are available today. We will be covering only selected leadership models under each of the four approaches.

Trait Approach

The earliest approach to the study of leadership concerned the personal characteristics of leaders. These attributes have been categorized as physical characteristics (age), background characteristics (education, social class), intelligence,
personality, task-related characteristics (achievement, need, initiative), and social
characteristics (supervisory ability, popularity) (Ivancevich et al., 1983). Even
though extensive research has been conducted in the area of personal traits, little
conclusive evidence has been gathered. As Robbins (1984) states: "Research
efforts at isolating these traits resulted in a number of dead ends (p. 334). Several
factors caused this lack of success (Ivancevich et al., 1983). The trait approach
ignored the employees or individuals being led and obviously they are a factor in the
leader's ultimate ability to influence behavior. Second, in most cases, the importance of the various traits has not been specified. This omission causes difficulty if
one must make a trade-off between a decisive or intelligent leader, for example.
Third, a problem resulted from the inconsistencies reported in the various research
efforts. Numerous contradictory statements regarding the positive or negative aspects of various traits resulted. Fourth, the list of traits continued to expand to such
a length that the process of choosing a leader would be made extremely difficult If
not impossible.

Behavior Approach

After failing to make much progress with the trait approach to leadership, researchers shifted toward trying to understand the behavior of effective and ineffec-

tive leaders. The interest became that of attempting to understand what leaders do or fail to do. Although several studies were conducted in this area, essentially all the studies focused on two features of leader behavior. One feature was the orientation toward accomplishing the job. The other feature was directed toward employees and satisfying their unmet needs. The two features can be summarized as follows:

> The people approach involves what the leader does to meet the individual needs of his or her employees. Behaviors here include such things as taking an interest in employee problems, smoothing friction among employees, and giving personal recognition. The task approach involves what leaders do to ensure the accomplishment of the group's work or task goal, and includes behaviors like setting performance goals, rewarding high performance, getting materials and supplies, and planning work. (Anderson, 1984, pp. 226–227)

While behavior might seem to be more relevant to understanding leadership than the leader's personal characteristics, conflicting results still existed. The attempt to determine the most effective leadership style was essentially abandoned and replaced by an approach that incorporates situational variables. As Schermerhorn (1984) states: "Indeed, most leadership theorists now recognize that the critical question is no longer which is the best style but really when and under what circumstances is a given style preferable to the others?" (p. 308).

Situational Approach

The approach to leadership receiving the most attention today is referred to as the situational, contingency, or reality based one. All these terms mean that the appro-

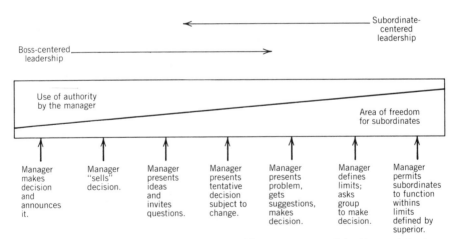

Figure 4.2. Leadership continuum. Reprinted by permission of the Harvard Business Review. An exhibit from "How to Choose a Leadership Pattern" by Robert Tannenbaum and Warren Schmidt (May/June 1973). Copyright © 1973 by the President and Fellows of Harvard College; all rights reserved.

priate leadership style depends on a number of factors. Rather than just saying "it all depends," managers have focused on trying to determine the particular set of variables on which "it all depends." To this date, no such list has been developed. Several approaches have received widespread recognition, and we will review one of the more popular situational leadership models.

One of the earliest, most popular, and easiest to understand of the models was developed by Robert Tannenbaum and Warren Schmidt (1980). It features a continuum, shown in Figure 4.2, that represents seven leadership styles ranging from the autocratic—"do it my way"—situation on the left to the situation on the right where more of a participative style is used. The height of the rectangle represents the authority relationship between the leader and the led. One can see that the authority focus shifts from the leader to the led as one moves from left to right on the continuum.

The three situational factors that should be assessed in determining which of the seven leadership styles is the most appropriate are the following:

- Forces in the manager
- Forces in the subordinates
- Forces in the situation

Forces in the manager include such factors as the leader's value system, confidence in employees, personal leadership inclination, and feeling of security in an uncertain situation. In motivational topics, we spend a considerable amount of time talking about how important employees are because they are individuals and have individual needs, drives, and desires. The same thing is being said here of the leader. Leaders are also different and have their own personal perspective, which they bring to a leadership situation. According to Tannenbaum and Schmidt (1980),

> The manager brings these and other highly personal variables to each situation he [sic] faces. If he can see them as forces which consciously or unconsciously influence his behavior, he can better understand what makes him prefer to act in a given way. And understanding this, he can often make himself more effective. (p. 289)

The second variable concerns issues at the employee level in contrast to the leader level. One example would be the need for independence and autonomy of the employees. If the employees have high needs for independence, all other things being equal, a leadership style toward the right of the continuum would be appropriate. Similarly, some employees desire to be told specifically what to do and others prefer more freedom. Other factors at the employee level are the employees' degree of interest in the problem, degree of shared organizational goals, and the amount of knowledge and experience that employees have in handling a particular kind of problem.

Certain features of the overall situation also affect the type of leadership behavior deemed appropriate. One such factor is the type of organization involved. There are many references to corporate cultures that are defined as the values, traditions, and beliefs that solidify an organization. Some organizatons focus more on the short-run "bottom line" and prefer their managers to be in control, decisive, and focused on key result areas. Other organizations place more emphasis on the long run and are more concerned about employees than the "bottom line." These different cultures suggest which supervisory behaviors are good or bad and, in turn, push a leader more toward one end of the continuum.

Another situational factor concerns how effectively the group members work together. If a group does not have an harmoniously united relationship, a leadership style toward the right end of the continuum may be risky. Another situational factor is the particular kind of problem. Some types of problems are handled better if input is received from group members, while other problems are best worked out by individuals in rather autocratic ways. The last situational factor is that of time available. If time is limited, the leader may have to make a decision and announce it. We should remember, however, the investment dimension of time. For instance, a leader may say something akin to the following: "I don't have time to bring Mary or Bob into decision making this time so I'll just go ahead and make the decision myself and save time." While such an approach may be in order on some occasions, the leader should remember that time wisely invested generates a return on that investment just like money does. In other words, even though time may be critical, an investment of time with employees may generate many returns in the future if they learn how to make better and more substantive decisions. In the short run, a leadership style on the right end of the continuum may seem to take more time but such may not be the case in the long run.

Tannenbaum and Schmidt (1980) have obviously not provided a rigid set of guidelines that can be plugged into some formula to arrive at the preferred leadership style. Two key benefits of their leadership model are the insight into the variables that really matter and the flexibility suggested by the leadership continuum. Autocratic leaders are not necessarily bad and participative leaders are not inherently good—"It all depends."

Another way to address a situational environment is outlined below and is similar to the three-factor approach above but might be a little easier to remember. We address this issue as follows: "In trying to decide on a leadership style, how do you answer the YES question?"

"Y" represents you the leader. What style is personally more comfortable for you? With which style have you had more success? With which style do you feel more security? The second letter—"E"—represents the employees being led. How long have you known them? What are their skill levels? What are their goals and needs? The third letter—"S"—stands for situational variables. How much time do you have? How much risk is involved? What style would my boss personally prefer?

Keep in mind the YES question as you try to handle the complexities of the leadership issues in management and supervision. While this leadership continuum is a popular approach, several other situational models also exist.

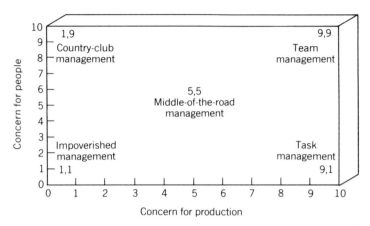

Figure 4.3. Managerial grid. Reprinted by permission of the Harvard Business Review. An exhibit from "Breakthrough in Organizational Development" by Robert Blake, Jane S. Mouton, Louis B. Barnes, and Larry Greiner (November/December 1964). Copyright © 1964 by the President and Fellows of Harvard College; all rights reserved.

Universal Approach

The last approach to leadership is referred to as the universal one. While most people subscribe to the situational approach to leadership, there are those who advocate a single style regardless of the situational factors. Probably the most widely known leadership model of this type is the Managerial Grid of Robert Blake and Jane Mouton (Blake & Mouton, 1978). The grid, shown in Figure 4.3, depicts "concern for production" and "concern for people." Each leader can be assessed somewhere along each axis using the one to nine scale. Even though there would be 81 cells on the grid, Blake and Mouton (1978) described five of the more significant ones as follows:

1. The 9,1 leader is primarily concerned for production and only minimally concerned for people. This type of leader, termed *task management,* believes that the primary leadership responsibility is to see that the work is completed.
2. The 1,9 leader is primarily concerned for people and only incidentally concerned for production. This type of leader, termed *country club management,* believes that a supervisor's major responsibility is to establish harmonious relationships among subordinates and to provide a secure and pleasant work atmosphere.
3. The 1,1 leadership style, termed *impoverished management,* is concerned for neither production nor people. This leader would attempt to stay out of the way and not become involved in the conflict between the necessity for production and the attainment of good working relationships.
4. The 5,5 leader reflects a middle-ground position and is thus termed middle-

of-the-road management. A leader so described would seek to compromise between high production and employee satisfaction.

5. The 9,9 leader's behavior is the most effective. This style, termed *team management,* is practiced by leaders who achieve high production through the effective use of participation and involvement of people and their ideas.

Even though Blake and Mouton suggest that the 9,9 style is the best one, there is little empirical evidence to substantiate this claim. Most people today say that the best leadership style is the one that fits a particular situation, and in that sense, "it all depends,"

SUMMARY

Leadership is an important topic for the supervisor because it impacts on performance and employee satisfaction. We have not yet learned all there is to know about leadership but we have made progress. The issue is not to try and identify the ideal leadership style but to become more aware of the contingency factors and to use the style that best fits a particular situation. Hopefully, the following points will assist you in furthering your understanding of leadership:

- Any style of leadership can be effective if it matches the requirements of a particular situation.
- Flexibility, yet consistency, is a key in an effective leadership style.
- First-level supervisors are the only managers who exclusively supervise non-managerial employees and this fact makes the leadership role unique.
- In the eyes of nonmanagerial employees, the supervisor often represents THE organization.
- The leader uses power to achieve results.
- The more effective leaders are aware of multiple power bases and how to use them.
- Some power bases derive from the organization and others are personal in nature.
- Power alone is not enough because the employee has to "accept" the request or directive.
- Leadership has been studied according to trait, behavior, situational factor, and universal approaches.
- Traits and behaviors have minimal use in predicting effective leaders.
- The three general situational factors, on which an effective leadership style depends, include you, the employees, and the situation (YES).

REFERENCES

Albanese, R., & Van Fleet, D. D. *Organizational Behavior*. New York: Dryden Press, 1983.

Anderson, C. R. *Management Skills, Functions, and Organization Performance*. Dubuque, IW: Brown. 1984.

Barnard, C. I. "The Theory of Authority." In Louis E. Boone & Donald D. Bowen (Eds.), *The Great Writings in Management and Organizational Behavior*. Tulsa, OK: Pennwell, 1980.

Blake, R. R., & Mouton, J. S. *The New Managerial Grid*. Houston: Gulf Publishing, 1978.

Flippo, E. B., & Munsinger, G. M. *Management*. Boston: Allyn & Bacon, 1982.

French, J. R. P., Jr., & Raven, B. "The Bases of Social Power." In Darwin Cartwright (Ed), *Group Dynamics: Research and Theory*. Evanston, IL: Row, Peterson, 1962.

Ivancevich, J. M., Donnelly, J. H., Jr., & Gibson, J. L. *Managing for Performance*. Plano, TX: Business Publications, 1983.

Likert, R. *New Patterns of Management*. New York: McGraw-Hill, 1961.

Robbins, S. P. *Management: Concepts and Practices*. Englewood Cliffs, NJ: Prentice-Hall, 1984.

Schermerhorn, J. R., Jr. *Management for Productivity*. New York: Wiley, 1984.

Schoen, S. H., & Durand, D. E. *Supervision: The Management of Organizational Resources*. Englewood Cliffs, NJ: Prentice-Hall, 1979.

Tannenbaum, R., & Schmidt, W. H. "How to Choose a Leadership Pattern." In Louis E. Boone & Donald D. Bowen (Eds.), *The Great Writings in Management and Organizational Behavior*. Tulsa, OK: Penwell, 1980.

Chapter Five

Controlling

Imagine a city with a population of approximately one million people. Further assume that the city had no traffic lights or stop signs. What would happen? We would have chaos because the traffic situation would be totally "out of control." Consider another situation where the same city installed traffic lights and stop signs at every intersection. What would happen in this situation? We would still have chaos because traffic would essentially be at a standstill but things are "out of control" for a different reason.

The point of the above example is that we cannot be effective supervisors unless we take a balanced approach toward control. Too few as well as too many controls will cause us problems. Such a perspective can be seen in Figure 5.1. In each case of too few and too many controls the result is the same—performance is not as high as it could be. The reasons for the poor performance are different. With too few controls, chaos and confusion led to the poor performance. Too many controls stifled initiative and led to stagnation.

It is important for us to see control as part of a process and not just an activity. We have observed that some people's orientation toward control can be summarized in statements such as the following:

> My job as a supervisor is to take charge of things when the situation gets out of control.
>
> I have to stay close to the people who work in my unit to make sure things stay under control.

Such statements do not reflect the proper perspective toward control as part of the supervisory process. These statements refer to only one activity that occurs in controlling—that of taking corrective action when and if it needs to be taken. In the next section, we will define control in terms of multiple steps. The effective supervisor is not one who merely "takes control," but one who also uses the control process.

The objectives of this chapter are as follows:

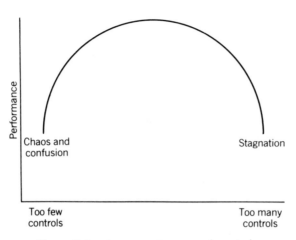

Figure 5.1. A perspective toward controls.

- To develop a vocabulary of control terminology
- To see control as a process and not just an activity
- To learn the various kinds of controls used by supervisors
- To learn the characteristics of effective control systems
- To understand how to handle control dysfunctions

DEFINITION OF TERMS

Control, which is part of the supervisory and management process, involves three essential steps:

- Establishing a standard
- Measuring and comparing against that standard
- Taking corrective action if necessary

The three steps are essential regardless of whether we are talking about budgetary control, materials usage control, quality control of patient care, or control of the human resources we employ.

The first step involves the establishment of some standard, benchmark, or target based on the goals and objectives established in the planning stage. In fact, control is really just the reverse side of the planning coin. In planning we establish goals and objectives, and through the control process we attempt to ensure that we are meeting or moving toward those goals and objectives. Some standards may be rather objective such as nursing hours per patient day. Other standards, such as maintaining employee job satisfaction or keeping the image of the hospital at a desired level, are less objective.

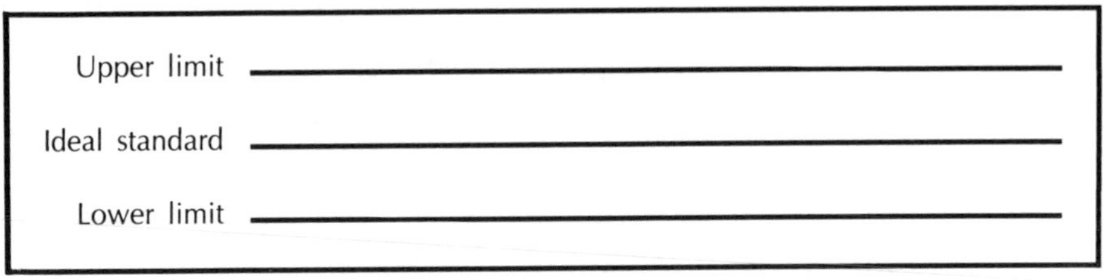

Upper limit ────────────────────────────────────

Ideal standard ────────────────────────────────────

Lower limit ────────────────────────────────────

Figure 5.2. Acceptable range of control measures.

The second step involves measurement of the item, process, or output that we are interested in and determining how that measure compares to the standard established in the first step. Supervisors typically measure performance by personal observation, statistical reports, oral reports, or written reports (Robbins, 1984). After the measure is obtained, a comparison is made to the standard. This comparison allows deviations from the standard to be detected. In many cases, a range of acceptable performance would be established around the standards so that measurements failing into that range would be acceptable. Assume, for example, that you are trying to control the number of nursing hours per patient day. As seen in Figure 5.2, some ideal standard has already been established. To think that such a standard can be achieved every day is far-fetched. You establish an upper limit because measures of nursing hours that exceed this limit might suggest that you are not being efficient. You also establish a lower limit because not reaching at least this limit may imply unsafe patient care. You then measure to see if you fall into the acceptable range. The third step results from the supervisory reaction to the measurement at step two.

In some cases, an acceptable range may not exist, and any deviation from the ideal would warrant supervisory attention. In other cases, no corrective action is taken unless the upper or lower limit is exceeded. This principle, however, must be modified through a number of points. One point is related to the trend effect. Using our nursing hours per patient day example, assume that you receive weekly reports regarding this area of interest. If the weekly reports that you have received for several weeks are similar to those plotted in Figure 5.3, you can obviously see a trend developing, which in all likelihood will lead to a case of exceeding the range of acceptable.

Even though your last several observations are technically within the range of acceptance, some additional attention or corrective action is needed. In another situation, you observe what is depicted in Figure 5.4. Observations for several weeks suggest that things are under control. The last observation is far different from those you typically receive. Again, technically speaking, the observation falls in the range of acceptance, although it is not typical. The observation could be significant and may need attention. A new term, *outlier,* has been adopted to describe this type of case. Outlier cases are as follows: ''Atypical hospital cases that have an extremely long or extremely short stay relative to most cases in the same Diagnosis Related Group'' (Medicare-Medicaid Guide, 1983). Obviously, the issue

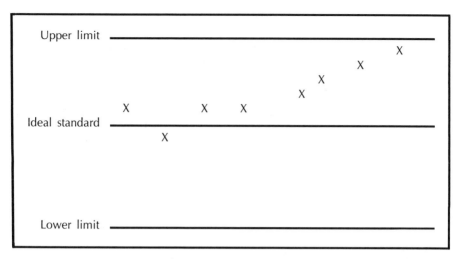

Figure 5.3. Trend effect.

is the same as the one we are describing in control processes. Control methodology continues to develop in the health care field.

In the preceding section, we stated that it is important to envision control as a process and not just a step of taking corrective action. When a situation appears to be "out of control," the underlying cause might be a result of any one of the three steps for establishing the standard, measuring and comparing, or undertaking the necessary corrective action. Suppose that in some operational area of the hospital, it is estimated that a particular unit of work should take an hour to perform if some ideal situation exists. You established a range of acceptance of ten minutes on either side of the ideal. Spending more than seventy minutes might mean that the employee is not efficient, and spending less than fifty minutes may mean that a thorough job is not being done. You receive reports that the task is repeatedly taking longer than seventy minutes. Rather than jumping to the assumption that the em-

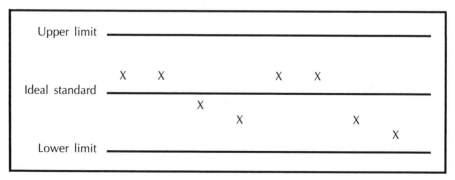

Figure 5.4. Outlier effect.

ployees are "goofing off" and you must do something to "bring things under control," you decide to examine the situation. You learn that some new procedures have been added to this area of work because of safety requirements. Because the unit of work around which the standard is formed has changed, perhaps your corrective action would consist of changing the standard. Hence, the focus of the change is at step one in the process and not just at step three. In some other situation, an erroneous written report that you receive indicates that the area is under control. After personal observation, however, you realize that some problems exist. The focus here is at the second step of measuring. What we are emphasizing is that supervisors need to think broadly about underlying causes of control problems.

Some of the key terms that we will be using in this chapter are defined as follows:

- *Preliminary control*—a "before the fact" focus on control.
- *Feedback control*—an emphasis on control during the time processes and events are occurring.
- *Control dysfunction*—some unintended consequence or reaction to a control measure.
- *Internal control*—a philosophy of control that assumes people can be trusted to maintain a sense of self-control.
- *External control*—a philosophy of control that assumes supervisors have to be there to keep things "under control."

BENEFITS OF SUPERVISORY CONTROL

Earlier we stated that management work is the activity associated with the functions of planning, organizing, staffing, directing, and controlling the efforts of individuals and the use of other resources to achieve individual, group, or organizational purposes. In planning, we emphasized the establishment of objectives. In organizing, we described how important the process of delegation is and how accountability must be established. In staffing, we covered the issues associated with acquiring and developing the necessary human resources to achieve objectives. In directing, we presented material related to leadership and motivational processes so that the efforts of the human resources would be aimed toward the goals and objectives we established in planning. Control, then, is the final link to ensure that these separate processes all fit together and that we do indeed make the intended progress.

There are other benefits associated with effective supervisory control (Boone & Kurtz, 1984). Control allows us to establish accountability. In order for people to be held accountable, they must understand what the expectations are, what standards of performance prevail, and how their performance will be measured and evaluated. This principle of accountability is at the heart of the delegation process, which is the initiating aspect of employee performance. Another benefit is that proper control processes allow us to be better prepared to handle change. When an organization is facing multiple, complex, and changing environments, effective controls allow for the detection of changes. A third benefit is that control measures better enable us to address the complexities of today's organization. Consider how hospitals are now becoming members of shared services systems or affiliates of major proprietory or international hospital companies, such as Hospital Corporation of America or Charter Medical Corporation. Controls provide mechanisms through which the effectiveness of the various units can be assessed. Controls are also beneficial because people do make legitimate mistakes. Sometimes the mistakes are small and at other times they are major. A properly designed control system will detect these mistakes and allow behavior and performance to be redirected.

Additional benefits accrue because control measures can be used in the following six areas (Boone & Kurtz, 1984).:

1. To make performance more consistent and standard so that efficiency prevails
2. To protect asset usage that might otherwise be abused through waste, theft, and misuse
3. To ensure that quality services and products are produced
4. To measure individuals' contributions
5. To assure that the organization's goals and objectives are balanced
6. To motivate people.

THE ROLE OF THE SUPERVISOR

The role of the supervisor is that same as that of any other executive or manager in the organization. At times, standards will be established by someone else in the organization and the supervisor measures, compares, and takes corrective action when necessary. At other times, the supervisor will be involved in all three steps of establishing, monitoring, and correcting situations. Supervisors would in general be responsible for controls in the area of quantity and quality of output, employee time usage in the production of those goals or services, and budgets.

Earlier we defined supervision and management as planning, organizing, directing, staffing, and controlling. Since directing is closely related to controlling, especially in the measuring and comparing phase, Figure 5.5 shows that first-line supervisors tend to spend more time on directing and controlling than on the other management functions.

ELEMENTS OF CONTROL PROCESSES

In an earlier section, we defined control in terms of three essential steps illustrating that control is a dynamic process and occurs over time. One way to further clarify the dynamic aspects of control systems as opposed to the static notion of merely "taking control" is to examine three types of control—preliminary control, concur-

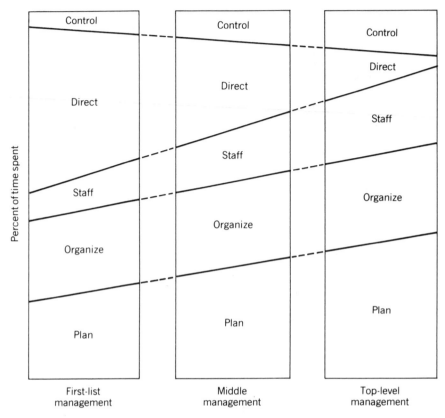

Figure 5.5.   Proportion of time spent on management functions by level of supervision.

rent control, and feedback control (Donnelly et al., 1984). In Figure 5.6, one can see that we have further clarified, through examples, preliminary, concurrent, and feedback control, and the items represented in that figure will form the basis for our discussion in the next several sections. Preliminary control measures are designed to handle our concern about physical, human, and monetary resources in a "before the fact" time frame. In other words, we would be attempting to determine before we purchased raw materials or before we hired employees that those resources met some predetermined standard. Obviously, the concern is to avoid having to later take corrective action because some resource did not meet standards prior to being used.

Concurrent control is the process through which activities and operations are monitored and directed. As can be seen in Figure 5.6, concurrent control involves the style of leadership that the supervisor uses in terms of directing operations and behaviors. Again, the concern is monitoring the processes so that activities do not become out of control and require extensive corrective action.

The focus in feedback control is one of "after the fact." Patients have been processed, monies have been expended, projects have been completed, and our

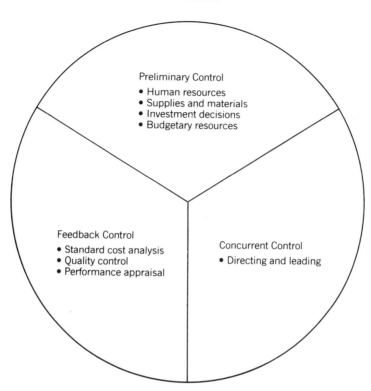

Figure 5.6. Preliminary, concurrent, and feedback control.

concern is to examine to what degree the earlier established standards were met. In general, feedback controls would have some type of unique time frame associated with them. For example, there may be daily, weekly, monthly, and even yearly reports that focus on events and activities "after the fact."

Another way to examine this time dimension of control processes can be seen in Figure 5.7. Regardless of whether one is supervising in a hospital, a clinic, or a long-term care facility, some type of "production process" is being used. We should remember that the term production process is not strictly associated with the production of tangible goods. For example, in hospitals where x-ray services are provided, one would still describe that service as a production process. In essence, inputs are used and through some process converted into outputs. Figure 5.7 provides further examples of inputs, processes, and activities used to produce outputs (various services or goods), and the control type associated with each.

Preliminary Control

If we think of control processes in terms of some type of a repetitive cycle, preliminary control would be focused on the front end of that cycle. As such, preliminary control is anticipatory in nature and attempts to ensure that the various types of

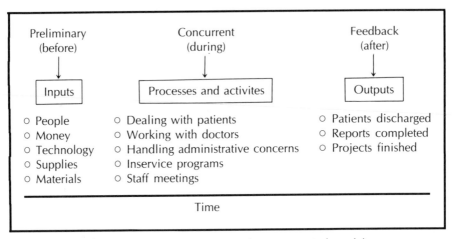

Figure 5.7. Input, process, and output control model.

resources required meet intended standards. In other words, thinking of our earlier production process whereby inputs are, through production processes, converted into outputs, we are trying at this stage to at least ensure that the inputs are the proper type even though things may become "out of control" during the production process or at the output stage. In this section, we will be describing various preliminary control issues associated with human resources, supplies and materials, investment decisions, and budgetary resources.

Human Resources

One type of resource obviously required in any organizational setting is people. Preliminary control regarding human resources would essentially involve those personnel procedures that are designed to ensure that only qualified human resources are being used. For example, a hospital may require that all registered nurses possess a baccalaureate degree. A long-term care facility may require that all housekeeping assistants have at least two years of experience. A drug abuse clinic may require three letters of recommendation for every person being considered for hiring. Health care organizations may also establish standards of a preliminary type to ensure that only various kinds of patients are admitted to the facility. Such standards may exist for reasons of economy and efficiency or may exist because of the lack of various technologies that would be used in such cases if they were admitted.

Supplies and Materials

Another area of preliminary control involves the various physical raw materials used in health care organizations. Medications, supplies, food, office materials, and linens are only a few of the areas in which some type of preliminary control would be established. Two concerns exist regarding the acquisition and use of these various supplies and materials: one issue is associated with the quality aspect of the goods and materials being received, while the other concerns the inventory levels. Let us consider an example of the first type in which our concern is associated with receiving only those supplies and materials that satisfy our quality standards. Suppose that a hospital uses an outside vendor to supply the various linens needed in the numerous aspects of the hospital. Initially, the linens received from this outside vendor were of a high quality and few problems were associated with the receipt of these linens. In time, however, the vendor's services began to deteriorate, and soiled and torn linens were occasionally being received. Let us further assume that we had no preliminary control measure established, and we began to use these linens in their soiled and torn states. Referring back to Figure 5.7, we can see that we are now moving in time from the input stage to the processes and activities stage. If we continue to use these linens in the soiled and torn states, the hospital would most likely have disgruntled and dissatisfied patients. In other words, we have now reached the output stage before we realize that we have a problem. A properly designed preliminary control measure would have detected the fact earlier that the linens were no longer of the desired quality, and action could have been taken at that stage.

The other concern regarding supplies and materials involves the level of inventories maintained. There is essentially a trade-off relationship to consider in this area of inventories. On the one hand, carrying excessive inventory levels depletes organizational resources and is not considered efficient. Operating capital is tied up, and the inventoried items may become obsolete, may be pilfered more often, and may spoil more frequently. On the other hand, maintaining excessively low inventory levels leads to a condition referred to as a *stock out* and perhaps interferes with the ability of the organization to provide the necessary services. Most organizations, therefore, establish some type of lower and upper limit regarding inventories to handle concerns of overstocking and understocking.

Investment Decisions

Investment decisions are different from expenditures. Expenditures typically represent relatively small amounts of money and in general the item purchased by the expenditure would have a short life span. We typically think of office supplies, spare parts and repair items, and operating supplies as expenditures. Investment decisions in most cases involve larger sums of money and the item purchased typically has a longer time frame. Although we often think of investment decisions in relation to equipment and facilities, we can also use the investment decision process in considering such things as new organizational models or new health care delivery models. Even though investment decisions, especially if they involve large sums of money, are usually made at the higher levels of health care administration, supervisors can still use the process in terms of considering investments at their own unit level, and they will often be asked for advice even though decisions will ultimately be made at higher levels. The primary concern in controlling investment decisions is to ensure that the organization receives an adequate rate of return on its investment. One interest is associated with the desire that the investment should at least cover its cost during its expected life span.

Suppose that you are the supervisor of the cafeteria in the hospital and are contemplating the purchase of a piece of equipment in the kitchen. That equipment is estimated to save you $2,500 yearly in salary and costs $10,000. The vendor estimates that the life span of the piece of equipment is three years. While this is an exaggerated example, it does make the point that the $7,500 saved ($2,500 for three years) does not equal or exceed the $10,000 invested and, everything else being equal, this would not be a good investment decision. Therefore, an organization may establish a preliminary standard that states that no investment decisions will be made if they involve a payback of longer than, hypothetically, five years.

A related concern is the return on investment that a particular investment decision generates. The principle here is the same as the one used when an individual decides to invest money in stock or bonds and is interested in choosing the highest rate of return qualified by the risk associated with the investment. In this case, an organization may establish a preliminary standard stipulating that no investment decision will be made that does not generate at least a 15 percent return on investment.

Supervisors and managers should also be aware of the issue of investment in human resources. For example, some people consider the management development of employees through seminars and workshops an expenditure of money. Such monies should be considered as investment because the payoff associated with such an expenditure is typically long run in nature. In other words, suppose that the hospital decides to spend $10,000 on a management development program to upgrade the skills of all its managers. The benefits received from such a program are in general not evident in the short run because it takes time to change people's attitudes regarding supervisory and management practices. Therefore, the money spent on such a program should be viewed as an investment in human resources. The same types of issues regarding return on investment should also be addressed here.

Budgetary Resources

In general, we use the term *budgets* in referring to financial resources, but budgets can also be associated with materials, time, and the usage of other resources. Obviously, the end consideration is associated with the monetary resource. Budgets are appropriate for consideration under preliminary control in that they are anticipatory in nature and attempt to spell out the needed financial resources prior to our entering into some process or activity. We would be at the beginning of an operational cycle when we began to use the budget.

Budgets would also define the various techniques and processes that would be used as we entered into the later stages of converting inputs through production processes into outputs. In other words, the budget would typically cover the type of equipment and number of people involved in conducting operations and as such would provide a general framework through which decision making would be implemented.

One last consideration associated with budgets is that budgets provide the framework through which managers are able to make decisions on their own without receiving the approval of higher authority (at least, that is the way budgets are intended to work). For example, when a supervisor is given the operating budget for her or his unit, it has been established in advance how much that supervisor is allowd to spend and, if a good management process has been followed, the supervisor may expend these monies without approval of higher authorities. Obviously, such a process involves delegation.

Budget controls should have the following characteristics (Schermerhorn, 1984):

- Strategic and oriented toward results
- Based on information
- Simple and understandable
- Prompt and oriented toward exceptions
- Flexible
- Based on controllable factors
- Fair and objective
- Positive and conducive to self-control

Concurrent Control

Directing and Leading

Concurrent control refers to the leadership style that the supervisor uses in trying to ensure that work performed falls within allowable standards. Earlier, we stated that supervisors plan, organize, staff, direct, and control. Direction and controlling are quite closely related. These latter two elements involve the various mannerisms, approaches to communication, and the methods in which the supervisor accomplishes the ''telling'' part of the supervisory role. Concurrent control would encompass the actual instruction that supervisors provide employees regarding appropriate procedures of work and the manner in which the work of the employees is overseen to ensure that it is properly performed. In an earlier chapter on direction, we discussed leadership style. Certainly, the manner in which a supervisor maintains concurrent control often depends on leadership style. Various leadership models have been discussed in Chapter 4, so only the highlights will be covered here in terms of maintaining concurrent control.

In large measure, the type of concurrent control that a supervisor uses is based on the assumption that the supervisor makes regarding human behavior. Douglas McGregor was one of the first to recognize this principle and labeled these behaviors as Theory X and Theory Y (McGregor, 1960). According to McGregor, a Theory X manager assumed that workers were lazy, indifferent to organizational goals, irresponsible, and as such would have to be controlled through the use of external measures. In other words, a Theory X manager assumed that people performed either to obtain rewards or avoid punishment. The style of leadership used in maintaining concurrent control in this situation would be one of close supervision, top-down communications, and a "staying right on top of things" approach. Some key attributes of such a leadership style would be those of monitoring, inspecting, watching, and checking.

A Theory Y manager would assume different ideas about people. A Theory Y manager would believe that people will contribute to organizational goals if given a chance and are capable of self-control and direction. As such, a Theory Y manager would exhibit much more of a "hands off" style of maintaining concurrent control. That supervisor would maintain control through what is referred to as internal means. An internal control philosophy is based more on the internal needs of individuals who desire a certain amount of freedom, autonomy, and independence and, in turn, can be allowed to control themselves. The supervisor's actions under such an approach would be more of coaching and counseling rather than watching and inspecting.

We should be aware that while Theory X sounds "bad" and Theory Y sounds "good," such is not the case. Under the right set of circumstances, a Theory X style of maintaining control is entirely appropriate. Similarly, in the wrong set of circumstances, a Theory Y style can cause problems. What we are describing is a situationally based approach to maintaining concurrent control.

Schoen and Durand (1979) specified six attributes of an effective external control system. First, the method of measuring performance should measure the complete job; otherwise, those activities that are not measured will not be controlled. The control measures should also be based on objective measurements and should be capable of influencing the employee. Second, performance standards should be mutually established. When performance standards are mutually determined, the employee is likely to be far more committed than if a one-way, top-down approach is followed. Third, if external control systems are to be effective, job performance should be monitored by both the employee and the immediate supervisor. This process allows the employee to receive rapid feedback regarding performance. Fourth, the employee and immediate supervisor should both receive information regarding the employee's performance. Fifth, the information collected regarding employee performance should be transmitted as quickly and as frequently as possible. Taking corrective action is made more difficult if the information is received too late or has become outdated. Lastly, external rewards should be those items that are preferred by the employee. While added pay might be valued by one employee, a more secure work environment would be preferred by someone else. It can in general be stated that no single reward is likely to please everyone to the same degree. Therefore, the effectiveness of the external rewards will vary depending on how employees value the various rewards used. Schoen and Durand (1979) suggest that such factors as pay, promotion, dismissal, praise from the supervisor, interesting work, tenure, and status are examples of external rewards and, therefore, are appropriate in external control systems.

While at times external control measures are appropriate, in other situations internal control systems are deemed more necessary; thus several conditions should be met as internal control measures are developed (Schoen & Durand, 1979). First, the measurement system should be complete and objective, just as is the case with

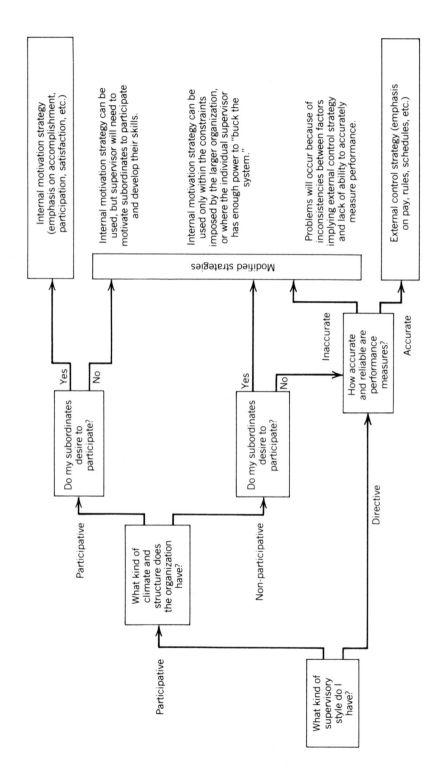

Figure 5.8. A decision tree for choosing a control strategy. (From S. M. Schoen, and D. E. Durand, *Supervision: The Management of Organizational Resources*, © 1979, p. 191. Reprinted by permission of Prentice-Hall, Inc., Englewood Cliffs, N.J.)

external controls. Second, the employee should be allowed to establish his or her own goals and standards and they should be of moderate difficulty. Obviously, in this case, the supervisor will still have some ultimate control, but the employee should experience the satisfaction that is associated with the added autonomy. Third, the employee should be allowed to monitor job performance. The underlying philosophy of an internal control system is one of trust and it would be inappropriate for the supervisor to exert a strong directing role here. Fourth, as with external controls, the information should be provided to the employee as soon as practical. Fifth, internal control systems are more feasible on jobs in which employees have a relatively high degree of autonomy. The employee should be able to identify more fully with the entire job when the feeling of "this is mine" prevails. Some of the situational factors that are relevant in choosing an internal or external concurrent control philosophy are described in Figure 5.8.

Our observations indicate that some supervisors think a participative style of control implies permissiveness. In other words, we are creating an environment in which employees will be allowed to "vote" on whether they want to perform or not. Such is not the case at all. In fact, we are describing the behavior pattern that the supervisor exhibits when providing instructions, correcting actions, and following up. A supervisor who uses an internal control philosophy is still in charge, still makes decisions, and still reserves the right to disagree with employees. The basic difference is the *style* used in the day-to-day contacts between supervisor and employee.

Feedback Control

Feedback control refers to actions taken after the fact and is based on an assessment of historical outcomes. Such information would be used in terms of adopting corrective actions for the future. For example, a monthly budget report received "after the fact" would provide information that the supervisor would use in terms of expenditures for upcoming periods. Feedback control is more advantageous than preliminary control and concurrent control for two reasons (Robbins, 1984). First, feedback control provides managers and supervisors with information regarding the effectiveness of planning. In other words, if the variation between the established goal and the reported results is minor, one would assume that the planning effort was appropriate. If the variation between the established goals and feedback performance measures is significant, most likely the new plans that would be developed would incorporate this feedback information and appropriate modifications would be included to make the plans more reasonable. Second, feedback control directly relates to employee motivation. People want to receive feedback on their performance and this information can obviously be conveyed in feedback control information. Although there are numerous examples of feedback control measures, we will discuss standard cost analysis, quality control, and performance appraisals as examples.

Standard Cost Analysis

Standard cost analysis is a process through which actual costs are compared to standard costs to determine any variances. If actual costs have exceeded standard costs, we refer to that situation as an unfavorable variance. And, if actual costs are less than standard, we call such a situation a favorable variance.

Standard cost analysis can be applied to supplies, overhead, labor, and almost any other category for which we can determine appropriate standards. We will limit our example to supplies only. Suppose that you are the supervisor in charge of the supply unit of a particular hospital. From historical data, you have determined that an average of eight scrub suits are used per operation in the hospital. Furthermore, these scrub suits cost five dollars each. After some specified time frame, you receive an expenditure report showing that $11,000 had been spent on scrub suits. Your feedback information further shows that 250 operations were conducted during that time frame. Standard cost analysis would suggest that $10,000 (250 $\times$ 8 $\times$ 5) should have been the amount spent for scrub suits. Obviously, in this case, we have an unfavorable materials variance of $1,000. As the supervisor of the unit, you would then begin to look for reasons that caused this variance. Perhaps the variance was caused by using more scrub suits than the standard, or perhaps the variance was caused by spending more per scrub suit than was used in the development of the standard. Such analyses and examinations would be undertaken with the expectation that corrective action would be implemented for upcoming periods of time.

Quality Control

Although quality control techniques can be used at the input and process stages of the production model, we will describe the quality control technique as part of the output portion of that model. The supervisory and managerial interest is one of ensuring that the various outputs produced possess the necessary characteristics that you earlier determined as appropriate. While the term *quality control* is usually used in the production of tangible goods, the concept is entirely appropriate in the production of services also. Therefore, we will use an example from the nursing division in a hospital.

Nurses in general would refer to this concern of quality control by the use of the term *quality of care*. The quality of the nursing care should be assessed in accordance with the following prioritized listing (Rowland & Rowland, 1980).

- Outcome
- Content
- Processes
- Resources
- Efficiency

The top priority regarding the type of nursing care received should be measured by the outcome of that care. This outcome measurement refers to changes that occurred in the health status of the patient. Positive examples of changes might include the following (Rowland & Rowland, 1980):

• An increase in health knowledge
• The ability to maintain positive health behavior
• The ability to function and work in personal roles

Examples of negative outcome measures might include the following (Rowland & Rowland, 1980):

• Failure to maintain health status
• Discomfort
• Disability
• Complications

In other words, the question being asked is, "Did the patient's health status change as a result of the nursing care received?"

Another type of quality of care concern is based on the content dimension. By an assessment of content, it is meant, "What did the nursing care actually 'contain'?" In this situation, the nursing care delivered would actually be assessed in terms of the various standards and procedures that were followed for a specific patient's situation.

The third type of quality of care assessment involves the various processes involved in rendering patient care. In this situation, we are examining the types of events occurring, the sequence, and the interaction with other components of the health care team.

Assessment of resources concerns "accessibility, availability, appropriateness, and acceptability" of the resources used in providing patient care (Rowland & Rowland, 1980).

The efficiency approach to quality of care is essentially one of cost benefit. The interest resides in determining whether the resources used in providing patient care were used in the least expensive manner.

In every one of these examples, the perspective is one of "after the fact", and the interest resides in determining whether the services delivered met some earlier determined standard. As such, we are still using feedback types of controls.

Performance Appraisal

Performance appraisal is usually viewed as a type of feedback control because the performance of employees is appraised after it has occurred. Such a perspective is only partially valid. In fact, performance appriasal should be seen as part of a process and not just some event that occurs after a person performs. We have witnessed situations in which some organizations believe that they have an effective performance appraisal system when they merely sit down after twelve months have lapsed and complete a form on an employee's performance. Rather, an effective performance appraisal system should include the following four steps:

1. Goals and objectives for the employee are clearly, objectively, and mutually determined.
2. Ongoing, direct feedback is provided to the employee regarding the positive and negative aspects of performance.
3. At a designated time, a specific, usually written, recording of prior performance is accomplished.
4. Desired performance is rewarded accordingly.

Several important comments must be made regarding these four steps. In the first item, the word "mutual" is emphasized as it relates to the determination of goals and objectives. Today's management literature contains many examples and benefits associated with participative approaches to decision making. Such a participative style is also used in the establishment of goals and objectives. As John Naisbitt (1982) suggests, "People whose lives are effected by a decision, must be a part of the process of arriving at that decision" (p. 59). The essential interest here is one of commitment. When employees are involved in and consulted during the decision-making process, as well as in the establishment of their own goals and objectives, they are far more likely to be committed to the ultimate goals and objectives delineated.

Another comment that should be made regarding the four-step process is the ongoing feedback that should be provided to employees. In our seminars on performance appraisal, we make the following statement: "There should be no surprises at performance appraisal time."

If a supervisor waits until performance appraisal review time to unload everything on an employee, the process is not likely to be nearly as effective as providing ongoing, immediate, and quick feedback as behavior is observed. In other words, when a supervisor finds an employee performing even slightly less than the intended goals and procedures, such behavior should be corrected immediately. By following such an approach, the employee does not go too far "off track." The situation with the employee would never become considerably "out of control", if the supervisor provides ongoing feedback.

The third step is undertaken to record officially the evaluation. At this time, new goals for the upcoming time period may also be discussed.

Lastly, if employees are responding to the challenges incurred by the establishment of goals, the performance should be rewarded appropriately. If the desired performance is not reinforced by rewards, the desirable behavior patterns are likely to change to undesired ones.

Numerous performance appraisal techniques and methods exist, and it is not our intent here to review those processes. It is important, however, that we view performance appraisal as a form of control. Returning to our basic definition of control in which we establish standards, measure, and implement corrective action when necessary, we can see that the same three steps are appropriate in terms of human behavior.

CHARACTERISTICS OF EFFECTIVE CONTROL SYSTEMS

In earlier sections, we indicated that controls include several types—preliminary control, concurrent control, and feedback control—that may be implemented using different styles—internal or external. Furthermore, any type of control should possess the following characteristics (Boone & Kurtz, 1984).

1. Controls should be clear and understandable. Performance is a function of motivation, skills and abilities, and role clarity. If controls are not clear and understood, a person does not have role clarity and we will not see the desired performance level. The person could be highly motivated and have the skills and abilities, but all three factors must be present in order to see the desired performance level.

2. Controls should be designed to match the activity under consideration. Information that has been collected should be appropriate for a particular activity. In other words, the maintenance department supervisor must receive information regarding the performance of people and activities in that unit. The housekeeping supervisor must receive information on housekeeping activities and personnel.

3. Controls should be developed so that deviations from standards are detected quickly. If adequate use is made of preliminary controls and concurrent controls, we should not experience extreme cases of substandard performance. Control systems should detect deviations early and suggest appropriate action by the responsible individual. Suppose, for example, the unit supervisor is responsible for some kind of output. In Figure 5.9 we will see that an ideal standard has been established with a lower and upper limit. Further assume that you have established a procedure that requires output to be measured at the close of work every Friday afternoon. On the first Friday indicated in Figure 5.9, your observations reflect the fact that even though output was slightly below standard, the situation was still within the acceptance regions. Even though you did not make observations on Saturday though the following Thursday, the actual situation that was occurring is depicted in Figure 5.9. On the next Friday, which is reflected on the right portion of the diagram, you determined that things are "out of control" and some managerial action is required. A control system that was designed to detect deviations more quickly would have prevented this occurrence.

4. Controls should be flexible. Any organization faces changes in environmental factors and certainly the health care industry is no exception. There are changes in the cost of raw materials, wage rates, shipping charges, and utility costs. Flexible controls are designed so that quick adjustments can be made when changes occur in these and other environmental factors.

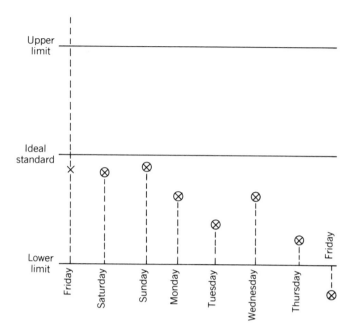

Figure 5.9. A faulty control system.

5. Costs incurred in implementing and maintaining control systems should be realistic. The cost of a control system should be compared to the benefits received from such a system. There are occasions when the monies expended on a control system might exceed any benefits to be gained by having the control system. Essentially, some type of a cost benefit analysis should be performed to ensure that the control system is the most economical one to accomplish the desired goals.

6. Control systems should prescribe corrective action. An effective control system not only identifies deviations from desired performance standards but also prescribes who should take corrective action and the area in which substandard performance is occurring.

7. Control systems should be effective and reflect reality and not be subject to manipulation. A poorly designed control system can be used by people to distort information and reflect situations unlike what is actually occurring. The more objective the control system is, the less likely such distortions can occur. Although supervision and management certainly contain many subjective aspects, performance should be measured on an objective basis (Boone & Kurtz, 1984).

CONTROL DYSFUNCTIONS

A control dysfunction is some unintended result as a consequence of a poorly designed control system. For example, if control measures are not flexible enough, are not timely enough, or are easily manipulated, people will occasionally "beat the system." Consider the following example, which is not from the health care sector but is relevant in terms of illustrating a dysfunctional principle:

> The city council in a large city in the midwestern part of the United States had implemented a control measure designed to limit the purchases of the unit managers in city government. The upper limit that a department head could spend without higher approval was $2,000. The supervisor of the Parks and Recreation Department submitted a request to city council for twenty golf carts each costing $1,500 and obviously giving rise to a total request of $30,000. At that time the economic signals were such that city council thought this was an excessive expenditure on something like golf carts and denied the department head's request. Shortly afterward the supervisor began to submit individual invoices covering one golf cart at a cost of $1,500. Obviously, he "beat the system" because, although the city council's intent was that the golf carts should not be purchased, he was still able to obtain the golf carts.

Suppose that you are a unit supervisor in a hospital and have established a control measure that basically counts inspections of some piece of mechanical equipment in the hospital. If the emphasis of the control system is merely counting inspections, the employees may conduct sloppy inspections merely to meet the quota.

Another example of a counterproductive or dysfunctional control system occurs in an agency where the supervisor is so concerned about employee attendance and performance that the supervisor initiates sign-in/sign-out control system. Every employee is required to sign-out and sign-in for both the morning break and the afternoon break. This overcontrol upsets the employees so much that they spend far more time at their desks complaining about the insult associated with signing-in and signing-out rather than concentrating on their work.

Using one measure, such as output, instead of many to evaluate performance will cause us to experience dysfunctional consequences. In other words, if we emphasize just output, people will pursue output at the sacrifice of other important areas of interest. If we emphasize good public relations, people will pursue public relations at perhaps the sacrifice of output. We need multiple standards that reflect the multiple interests.

Dysfunctions can also occur whenever people manipulate control data. Budgets represent an area in which people at times manipulate data merely to look good. For example, expenditures might be delayed in one month so that they fall into the beginning of next month and the control system will not detect such manipulations. In another area, a budget has been established with operating supplies, equipment, and capital expenditures as categories. In some situations when operating supplies run low, the equipment budget might be used to cover this shortage. In similar areas, we are describing various "games" that people at times "play" to avoid detection by the control system. It is extremely important that our earlier discussed characteristics of effective control systems be used to avoid such dysfunctional consequenses. Control measures, if properly developed, should be seen by operating supervisors and managers as an intergal and important part of a management system and not some device that is to be manipulated or distorted.

PLANNING AND CONTROL SYSTEM: MANAGEMENT BY OBJECTIVES

Earlier we stated that control is the opposite side of the planning coin. As we are pursuing the planning process, we establish various goals and objectives. As we move forward through time, we attempt to ensure that those goals and objectives are met. One technique that is available for integrating these two parts of management is management by objectives (MBO). MBO is a participatory approach to objective setting between supervisor and employee. Most MBO programs have a set of steps similar to the following (Boone & Kurtz, 1984):

1. Employee develops a description of performance areas and discusses this description with the supervisor.
2. Short-term performance standards are developed.
3. The supervisor and employee occasionally meet to discuss progress or lack of progress toward the achievement of the established goals and objectives.
4. Specific periodic dates are established at which the supervisor and employee will discuss progress.
5. At the end of the agreed on period, the supervisor and employee meet to evaluate progress and to establish a new set of goals and objectives for the next time cycle.

Several features of an effective MBO model are worthy of additional comment. One required characteristic is that the goals and objectives be established jointly between supervisor and employee. When the employee participates in the establishment of goals and objectives, there is a greater commitment to them. The employee knows what must be accomplished and how evaluation will occur.

One can see that there are several specific parts of an MBO program that involve control. It is not important to try to separate the steps in an MBO program as planning versus control, but to see that control in and of itself means nothing. Control is only appropriate if it relates to the achievement of goals and objectives established in the planning stage.

HOW TO MANAGE CONTROL

Almost everyone today approaches management from a situational perspective. Such a perspective means that few absolutes exist in management and what we do as supervisors and managers will depend on a particular situation. Since such a perspective is appropriate for the entire management process, it must furthermore be appropriate for control processes. In the following sections, we will describe several factors on which a particular control system depends (Robbins, 1984).

Size of the Organization

As an organization expands, its control systems become more formalized and, in turn, perhaps impersonal. Small organizations can operate on informal rules and procedures or mere word-of-mouth practices. Obviously, larger organizations require more consistency and resort to more written and objective control systems.

Position and Level in the Organization

Jobs at lower levels in organizations typically have clearer definitions of performance standards that make the objective measurement of output more possible. As one moves higher in the organization, the control systems tend to be based on multiple criteria. This tendency reflects the broader range of interest of people higher in the organization.

Degree of Decentralization

If an organization is highly decentralized, the need for feedback controls will be greater than in situations in which the organization is highly centralized. If the authority in a highly centralized organization rests essentially at the top, the need for feedback controls is less than it would be in a decentralized organization.

Culture of the Organization

Some organizations have a climate where trust, openess, sharing, and communications are highly visible. Other organizations, however, foster a sense of threat, reprisal, fear, and intimidation. In the first organization, the control style would tend to be based more on internal measures, while in the latter organization the control system would be based on external measures.

Importance of an Activity

If an activity is so important that even a minor mistake can be extremely costly and create tremendous problems, a significant and extensive control system is necessary. However, if an activity is not so important and, furthermore, if controlling that activity is costly, a control system that is not so elaborate will probably be developed.

SUMMARY

Control is an essential part of management and is closely related to the planning process. In planning, goals and objectives are established and controlling allows for progress toward goal achievement to be assessed. The following points should facilitate the development of a proper control perspective.

- Control is more than just "taking control." Control is a process that involves the establishment of standards, measurement comparison, and taking corrective action if necessary.

- There can be just as many problems associated with having too many controls as there are with having too few controls. What we try to achieve is some degree of balance among the number, type, and extent of controls that we establish.
- How we implement a control process is primarily a matter of style. One type is referred to as internal control and relies more on trust and respect for the individual. The other type is referred to as external control and relies more on the offer of rewards or the threat of punishment.
- There are various types of control. Preliminary control concerns resources and activities before the fact. Concurrent control primarily concerns how we direct and lead employees and occurs at the same time performance is taking place. Feedback control occurs after the fact and uses historical information as a guide for making future decisions.
- There can be dysfunctions or unintended consequences associated with controls. We need to be sure that we do not overdefine controls, build controls that are too rigid, establish controls that do not allow for environmental changes, or develop controls that can be manipulated.
- Even though the word control at times may convey negative ideas, there is nothing wrong with having good control systems. There are numerous benefits associated with maintaining managerial control.
- The first-line supervisor is in general the most visible individual in an organization who handles control processes, especially in terms of directing and guiding employee activities.

REFERENCES

Boone, L. E., & Kurtz, D. L. *Principles of Management*. New York: Random House, 1984.

Donnelly, J. H., Gibson, J. L., & Ivancevich, J. M. *Fundamentals of Management*. Plano, TX: Business Publications, 1984.

McGregor, D. *The Human Side of Enterprise*. New York: McGraw-Hill, 1960.

Medicare-Medicaid Guide. Chicago: Commerce Clearing House, 1983.

Naisbitt, J. *Megatrends*. New York: Warner Books, 1982.

Robbins, S. P. *Management: Concepts and Practices*. Englewood Cliffs, NJ: Prentice-Hall, 1984.

Rowland, H. S., & Rowland, B. L. *Nursing Administration Handbook*. Germantown, MD: Aspen, 1980.

Schermerhorn, J. R. *Management for Productivity*. New York: Wiley, 1984.

Schoen, S. H., & Durand, D. E. *Supervision: The Management of Organizational Resources*. Englewood Cliffs, NJ: Prentice-Hall, 1979.

PART THREE

ESSENTIAL SKILLS FOR EFFECTIVE HEALTH CARE SUPERVISION

Chapter Six

Communication

Supervision is often described as the practice of producing results through people. Few would disagree. As we discussed in both Chapters 1 and 4, the major part of a supervisor's job involves directing the efforts of others. It is impossible to do this without communicating. Likewise, it is impossible to fulfill any of the functions of management, such as planning, organizing, staffing, directing, or controlling, without communicating. Many other facets of a manager's job, such as being able to coordinate with other work groups and dealing with the environment, could not be done without communication.

Of all the skills necessary to be effective in supervision, communication is probably the most important. It is the enabling process that allows information to be transferred and ideas to be translated into action. Perhaps the best way to look at communication from a supervisory perspective is to first understand and analyze the processes that exist when two people communicate with one another.

INTERPERSONAL COMMUNICATION DYNAMICS

The simplest way to analyze the interpersonal communication dynamics that exist between two people is to first look at one person as a sender and the second person as a receiver. For communication to occur, the message must be transmitted from a sender to receiver. Before the message is even transmitted, however, a number of factors enter into the communication process. The first factor involves the consideration that both sender and receiver are unique people. They have different personalities, different needs, different values, and, most important, different feelings, which often drive the dynamics of much of the communication process. No matter who these two people are, whether they are closest friends, worst enemies, close relatives, least preferred co-worker, best boss, or whomever, they will have different needs, values, and feelings that will drive their communication processes.

Many times the communication process deteriorates before it reaches the message transmittal stage because the person who is sending the message codes the

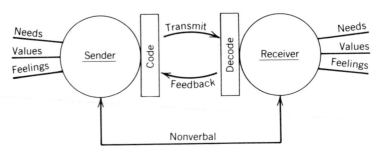

Figure 6.1   The communication process.

message improperly. Because we cannot transmit messages straight from one mind to another, it is essential that the message be translated into a language that allows it to be sent to the receiver. We call this a coding process. People often do not code properly. We have often heard people state: "That's not what I meant." Or: "I didn't mean to say that." Or: "I think you misunderstood." Usually these responses are symptoms of faulty coding by the sender. The message is then transmitted using the coded symbols that the sender has chosen, and it must then be decoded by the receiver.

The receiver's decoder is most likely different from the sender's coder. Our coding and decoding mechanisms have developed as a result of our training, experiences, background, and the kind of skills we develop. Therefore, it is often the case that a receiver will hear the same words and attach to them a different meaning.

This is one reason many people believe there is no such thing as effective one-way communication. For communication to be effective, there must be a feedback loop associated with the process. For example, many senders, rather than ask, "Did you understand?", will ask, "What did you understand?" The purpose is to hear in the receiver's own words that person's interpretation of the meaning of the message. A more comprehensive communication model than this one considers the coding mechanisms, decoding mechanisms, message transmittal, and feedback loop, as illustrated in Figure 6.1.

One further complication that adds still another significant dimension to the communication process is the dimension of nonverbal communication. While information is being transmitted back and forth on a verbal level, significant information and meaning are being simultaneously transmitted on a nonverbal level. The information that is transmitted on a nonverbal level can be even more significant than the verbal information in giving true meaning to the sentence. Thus, for a person to be a truly effective listener, it is important that the person listen to and observe the total communication process, both verbal and nonverbal (Haney, 1973).

Thus, to optimize communication skills as both sender and receiver, a supervisor should clearly understand these critical elements of communication, including the following:

1. Sender and receiver are unique personalities. They have different needs, values, and feelings. They also have different skills, knowledge, and experiences that will have an effect on their communication skills.

2. For a sender to send a message, it must first be coded. The sender's coding mechanism and ability to articulate is based on the sender's background, experience, and training.

3. Before the message can have meaning to the receiver, it must be decoded. The receiver's decoder will always be different from the sender's coder. Sometimes the difference may be significant, and other times it may not be. It is important to know that the decoding process occurs in a place other than in the coding process.

4. The receiver then interprets the message on the basis of his or her needs, values, and feelings.

5. Feedback is essential. For communication to be effective—that is, the sender should be able to rely on the fact that the message was received—feedback must occur.

6. Nonverbal communication is always present and can be as important as the verbal aspects of the communication process.

Another factor that affects the dynamics of the interpersonal communication process is the rate at which we speak and the rate at which we think. The average person in typical Western culture communicates at a rate of approximately 120–125 words per minute. The average person thinks at a rate of approximately 4–5 times as fast. This raises concerns for both senders and receivers. Senders must learn to send in concise information packages. They should place the important information at the front of each sentence, and the senders should ensure that they take steps to keep the receiver with them. They do not want the receiver to be too far ahead in the listening process since confusion will be the result. Receivers have an equally important issue to consider. Receivers have excess air time that must be managed properly. Use this excess air time to evaluate the content of what is being said, to ponder nonverbal information that is being transmitted, or to assess the sincerity of the sender's message. Receivers can also use this excess air time to think up a response. However, if the receiver spends too much time trying to think up a response, it is likely that much of what the sender is transmitting will be missed and interruptions will occur. With this framework in mind, it is worthwhile to understand in greater detail what some of the issues on both the sending side and the receiving side are likely to be in the context of the supervisor's role. Next we will discuss sending skills, receiving skills, and the creation of an environment for good organizational communication.

Sending Skills

Several different areas of the supervisory function rely on effective sending skills. Each of these areas, however, is characterized by different objectives. Since the objectives are different, the approach will be different and the factors that will operate in these different settings will vary from situation to situation. Four of these areas are as follows:

1. *Giving directions.* Although Chapter 4 discussed directing skills, here we will specifically examine a few of the communication guidelines for giving effective directions. In explaining the technique for giving directions, we are referring to a situation in which problems do not exist but performance is required and the supervisor is responsible for providing adequate instruction so that the desired performance can be achieved.

2. *Confronting.* This approach is used when an employee is performing inadequately or breaking the rules. It may also arise when a supervisor or someone higher up in the organization is creating a problem. Confrontation may also be necessary when a patient or someone from another department or someone from outside the organization is behaving in a way that is unacceptable. In these situations, confrontation will be relied on to correct the behavioral discrepancy.

3. *Giving presentations.* Formal presentations have become a necessity in modern day organizations. Presentations can be made to the hospital board for new equipment purchase, to the medical staff to implement new procedures, and to community interest groups about some new aspect of the organization's operations. Whenever the health care supervisor is requested to make presentations, credibility will be on the line. A person's credibility in an organization is determined by how well he or she conducts himself or herself in a formal communication setting such as in a presentation.

4. *Corresponding in writing.* Written correspondence is an integral part of today's organization. Although no one appreciates paperwork for the sake of paperwork, the fact is that without effective written communications, our organizations would not be able to operate. It is imperative today that supervisors at all levels be able to communicate clearly in writing.

These four areas, because of their special significance and importance in health care organization functioning, will be addressed separately in the following sections.

Giving Directions

As mentioned in several other chapters, giving directions is the primary responsibility of the health care supervisor. Directing is the main link in the chain of responsibility. It is at this level that ideas, goals, and objectives are translated into results. Therefore, it is essential that if the correct results are to be achieved, the directions must be precise, clear, well-timed, understood, and, most important, acted on correctly. This is a tremendous responsibility to place on the shoulders of the health care supervisor. It is important when shouldering this responsibility to give detailed attention to the communication processes associated with fulfilling this function. The following guidelines will help improve directing communications.

First Think Through What You Wish to Accomplish. A mistake many supervisors make is in responding to an impulse or a need, a feeling that certain communication is required, without thinking through the specific facets of that message that needs to be sent. As a result, from the time the need for the message is felt until it is coded, there is room for confusion. To minimize the possible errors that can be programmed into the message, it is worthwhile for the supervisor to first think through the message and determine the best ways to code the message so that the message that is intended is, in fact, the one that is sent.

The supervisor should pause before speaking to reflect on the information that is being used as a basis to formulate the message. The supervisor should determine the extent of action that is necessary on the part of the person who will be receiving the message and consider that different people might be targets for different objectives or different communication messages. For example, consider the charge nurse who is dissatisfied with the cleanliness of a particular work area. The nurse's objective is to have that area cleaned up and to maintain ongoing standards of cleanliness in the future. It is insufficient for that charge nurse to approach everyone who works in the area and simply state: ''This area is not clean enough. I would like it cleaned up and henceforth kept clean.'' Each person in the group has different responsibilities toward maintaining the cleanliness of that work area. Each person in the group has different perceptions of the extent to which they should contribute to its cleanliness. Thus it might be more effective for the charge nurse to say something such as, ''I'm dissatisfied with the cleanliness of this area and I would like steps taken to clean the area and I would like it to be kept cleaner than this in the future. Person A, specifically I would like you to follow through in this area; person B, your responsibilities will include the following; and person C, you will have still different responsibilities that include the following.'' If the charge nurse elaborates on what each specific responsibility is, everyone will now have a clearer understanding of what work he or she must do, how to do it, and how each person's work fits with the other members of the work group. In such a case, the work that is likely to be accomplished will be more efficient and more effective than with the overly general communication used in the first example.

Determine the Best Way To Communicate.   In the area of communication, we tend to develop repetitive habits. Sometimes these habits are useful because it helps people set expectations about how they are likely to hear from us. However, because communication situations and objectives can vary from circumstance to circumstance, this can also be a hinderance to effective communication. The supervisor who only passes out information during a monthly staff meeting or a weekly staff meeting is probably being inefficient in certain areas, because not all information is best transmitted through the form of a regularly scheduled staff meeting. The supervisor who communicates only after encountering a person in a chance meeting in a hallway or in some other work setting is probably not being efficient. The supervisor who relies only on written communication will suffer tremendous inefficiencies in the area of communication, as will the supervisor who relies only on the grapevine. All these different channels of communication and the modes that are associated with using them are more or less effective depending on the specific objectives that exist for a particular situation.

After thinking through your communication objectives, it is extremely beneficial to think through what is the best way to communicate your message to accomplish the desired objective. For many messages that a supervisor would like to send, many different modes will be employed. The modes are determined by the characteristics or the nature of the receiver as much as they are determined by the characteristics of the message itself. It is important to determine which modes people respond to for different kinds of messages and to develop a communication strategy that optimizes your effectiveness in light of that information.

Appeal to the Interests of Those Affected.   One problem with one-way communication is that it often ignores the interests, values, and perceptions of the people who are receiving the direction. Imagine receiving an advertisement from a major drug manufacturer for their new vitamins. Suppose the ad asked you to buy their vitamins because the company was having problems competing with all the new generic drugs on the market. The ad pressured you to buy because the company was having trouble paying its employees, covering expenses, and maintaining market share. Would that kind of message inspire you to buy their vitamins? It probably would not for most people. That is why the messages you receive are worded from a completely different perspective. The messages stress the positive effects of the vitamins on you and your health. The company talks about how good you will feel and how healthy you will be—factors that appeal to your personal self-interest.

Far too often, when communicating with people on the job, we ignore the interests of other people and we pay the price when we communicate in that context. It is essential when giving other people directions or communicating with them in ways we hope will inspire them to act in certain ways that we appeal to their values and interests and that we acknowledge factors in the situation that are important to them.

Give Feedback when Others Communicate to You.   When we are in a directing mode, we tend to fall into the trap that the supervisor is completely the sender and everyone else is completely the receiver. Senders receive too. It is important for people on the receiving end to be able to recognize that the input they are proposing is being considered. Receivers also have a need to be heard. Therefore, even though as a supervisor in a directive mode the primary emphasis is on sending, the supervisor must also be willing to listen, and listening means providing feedback to the other person to let him or her know that the message has been heard. It is difficult to influence another person when the sender is not open to influence. To encourage other people to remain open to influences, it is important that we as supervisors also remain open to influence.

Elicit Feedback on the Messages that You Send.   There is no such thing as effective one-way communication. Good supervisors don't ask, ''Did you understand?'' They ask, *''What did you understand?''* Feedback is the best method we have to combat confusion, misinformation, and misunderstanding. The only way we can be effective with it is to use it. It is important that we use this tool in virtually every communication setting that we find ourselves in.

Test the Effectiveness of Important Messages before Using Them.   No matter how careful we are, the same words mean different things to different people. It is usually worthwhile to test a message once it has been created. Choose several different people in several different work settings that are more likely to have different values and different needs. Present the message to them and elicit their feedback and the response they might have regarding the message's impact on them. Ask how they would respond to it, what problems the direction might create for them, and how they might word it differently to make the message more effective. Once the test is accomplished and the necessary corrections have been made, transmit the message on a broader scale to more people.

Provide Reinforcement, then Follow-up.   Imagine how confusing the world would be if we could say things only once and had to live forever with the consequences of our initial message. The result would be chaos and confusion. It is important, therefore, that every supervisor be ready and willing to repeat directions using different language or a different format and to follow through to whatever extent necessary to ensure that the directions are carried out. We do not live in a one-shot world and organizations are not one-shot environments. Organizations are multiple-shot environments that require multiple statements of the same directions to ensure effectiveness.

Confronting

Confrontation skills differ from directing skills. Directing skills are used usually in the absence of a problem when it is necessary to tell people how to do something, what to do, or what is needed. Confrontation skills are used when problems arise. These problems usually center on the behavior of one or more individuals. The behavior may be that of a member of the work group, a mid-level administrator, someone from another department, or someone from outside the organization. An important point to remember regarding confrontation skills is that the basic elements of a confrontation are to be used regardless of the relationship between the person who is doing the confronting and the person who is being confronted. Supervisors should use the same skills in confronting a subordinate as would be used to confront someone higher up in the organization.

An important factor in confrontation is power. People who have positional power in organizations are often the only ones who use confrontation. More often than not, anyone who confronts uses his or her positional power as a basis for achieving effective confrontation. The techniques we will discuss here are techniques that *do not* rely on positional power as a basis for effective confrontation. Personal power is a more viable basis for effective confrontation in today's health care organizations. If we develop the skills to confront unacceptable behavior on the basis of personal rather than positional power, we will be more effective in a wider variety of circumstances and hopefully will achieve better interpersonal relationships and more effective working relationships among co-workers.

Another concept to consider when talking about confrontation skills is the concept of assertive versus aggressive behavior. Different people have different needs. Aggressive people, for example, do what is necessary to satisfy their own needs without regard for the needs of other people. Assertive people, however, have their own needs met but also allow the needs of other people to be met as well. Our emphasis here is on being assertive rather than aggressive. We do not want to compromise our own needs as supervisors, but in satisfying our needs, we do not want to discount the needs of the other people we must work with. The following guidelines for devising assertive confrontations is adapted from Bower and Bower (1976).

Effective confrontations contain four elements: (1) a description of what happened; (2) a statement of the adverse effect of this action on the person or surroundings; (3) specification of some alternative ways to behave; and (4) an elaboration on the consequences of either changing or not changing. We will detail each of these points separately and analyze them to determine why each is an essential part of an effective confrontation.

To illustrate best how these four factors are used in designing an effective confrontation, consider the following example. A shift supervisor in an acute care facility is told by your supervisor (that is, by the administrator to whom you report) on Monday that effective at the beginning of next month all personnel under your supervision will be required to wear light yellow colored uniforms to conform with the hospital's new uniform standards. Further assume that on Wednesday the same person announced that effective the first day of the following month everyone of your shift would be required to wear brown plaid uniforms to work each day to conform with the company's new policy on dress. Now assume it is Friday, just prior to the weekly staff meeting, and you are confused regarding what the guidelines should be. On the one hand, you recall Monday's directions for yellow uniforms, and on the other hand, you recall Wednesday's directions for brown plain uniforms. What has happened in this situation is that the behavior of your supervisor has caused problems for you. This calls for a confrontation. Each of the four factors in an effective confrontation will be examined as they would be used in an example such as this one.

Describe the Event or Actions First.   Emphasis here is on the use of the word describe. Avoid interpreting the behavior and avoid drawing conclusions about the person from his or her behavior. Do not talk about the person or his or her personality. Do not talk about your conclusions about his or her personality on the basis of behavior: for example, an ineffective confronter might say, "You're a liar." Imagine the impact this would have on the receiver. The receiver will feel more defensive, resistant, and will automatically be placed in an argumentative positions. No one likes a label or personality characteristic handed down to them. The defensiveness and the barriers to communication happen because the receiver is immediately placed in a defensive position. The receiver feels angry about being called a liar or being called anything that reflects negatively on him/her as a person. Interpreting the behavior in a negative context as in this example saying, "you lied to me," is not much different from calling the person a liar.

If we simply want to follow the guidelines to describe the behavior, what would we say? Suggestion: "On Monday you told me all the uniforms should be yellow beginning the first of the month, and on Wednesday you told me all the uniforms should be brown plaid on the first of the month." Then stop—say nothing more. Consider now what is likely to happen. What are the likely responses from someone who receives this type of message? The most obvious response is for the person to reply with something such as, "Oh, you're right. I can see why you're confused. Let me clarify what I meant," and then they'll probably continue with an explanation that solves the problem. Another possible response is, "No, that's not what I said." In this case the sender simply says, "O.K., maybe I misunderstood. If you'll clarify it for me I won't have a problem." Again the problem will be solved. In some cases, however, the sender sends the simple descriptive message, and the receiver responds with something like, "Yes, that's right." Although there is agreement regarding a specific event or behavior that has caused a problem for the sender, that problem is not obvious to the receiver; therefore, it is necessary to proceed to the second step in the confrontation process and discuss the second factor.

Express the Effect on Me.   At this point, the sender explains why what happened is a problem *for the sender*. It is important to realize that if the behavior or the event was a problem to the receiver, we would not be at step two. If the behavior was a problem to the receiver, the receiver would not be doing it. It is the sender's problem, because the sender cannot accept the unacceptable behavior. Many ineffective confronters fail to realize this critical point. At this stage, they will say to the receiver: "You have a problem," when this happens. This response causes an immediate communication breakdown because the receiver perceives no problem.

Thus, to follow through with our example, at this stage of the process it would be appropriate for the sender to say something such as, "On Monday, you told me yellow, on Wednesday you told me brown plaid, now it's Friday morning and I want to tell the rest of the staff what to wear and I'm confused. I don't know what to tell them." Thus the emphasis in this message is placed on self: "I am confused" and "I don't know what to do." None of the emphasis in this portion of the message is on the receiver. None of the phrases begins with the word "You" and nothing in the phrases implies blame or transference of cause to the receiver. This is critical. In fact, many people who teach confrontational skills say that these first two elements are the only elements necessary for an effective confrontation. Dr. Thomas Gordon, author of Parent Effectiveness Training, defines these as "I messages" (Gordon, 1970). The emphasis in these messages is on one's self, the sender. In other words, when this happens, "I" am affected this way. In complex organizations, such as those we encounter in the health care field, however, it is probably not valid to assume that these first two steps will work in all confrontational settings. Although they will work in approximately 75 percent of the cases, there will be times when additional impact is required. This leads us to the next two steps.

Specify Alternatives.   Assume that, if the receiver has not responded satisfactorily until this point, part of the problem may be that the receiver has no idea how to act differently. Specifying alternatives means offering possible suggestions for the receiver to consider. Note the use of the word specify. This does not mean it is right for the sender to impose alternatives or to persuade the receiver forcibly. At this stage, it is important to communicate different ways of behaving that are acceptable without trying to impose our solutions on the receiver. The choice of whether to respond still belongs to the receiver.

Continuing with our example, then, some alternatives to consider might be as follows: "Would you care to specify one color or the other?" "Should I assume that the most recent instruction is the most valid?" "Unless I hear differently from you, I'll tell them brown plaid." In each of these cases, we are simply suggesting ways to behave that are acceptable to us, the sender.

Once again, in a small percentage of cases, this process may still not be adequate so, closely following the third step, we must employ the fourth strategy. The third and fourth steps, that of specifying alternatives and elaborating on consequences, usually fit closely together.

Elaborate on Consequences.   Consequences can be either positive or negative. Most of the time it is best to use positive suggestions and positive consequences. Negative consequences tend to sound threatening and are more difficult to handle. Consequences should be closely tied to the proposed courses of action. For example, when we specify alternatives as we did in step three, we would also want to include an explanation of the consequences that might arise from the different proposed courses of action.

In our example, this method might sound as follows: "If you definitely tell me which color of uniform to use, I can give the correct information at my weekly staff meeting." Specifying an alternative in this case offers the proposal to identify the desired color. The consequence, in this case a positive one, concerns being able to spread the word on time so people can act on it. An example of the same alternative with a negative consequence would be as follows: "If you don't tell me what color has been selected, then I won't be able to notify people of the change at our meeting this week." The alternative is still to clarify the information; the consequence in this case, however, is negative. The supervisor will not be able to achieve the sender's goal without adequate information to act on.

It should be noted in cases like this one that threats and coercive statements do not constitute specifying alternatives and elaborating on consequences. For example, if we approach a person and say, "Approve this request or I'll quit," this statement does not fit our confrontation mode. In this situation, we are trying to impose our will on the other person rather than allow that person the choice to act responsibly on our behalf. The difference is in providing the person on the receiving end with a free choice to respond in accordance with our needs and stated concerns. Threats tend to sound imposing.

Several people who teach confrontational skills believe these four steps are all that are required to achieve results and, although the addition of these last two steps will significantly increase our performance in confrontational situations, they will not guarantee success. Whereas use of the first two steps alone will probably work in about 75 percent of the cases we encounter, these last two steps will add another 20 percent. But in five percent or less of the cases in which confrontation is required, these skills will not be effective. In these cases, the supervisor has two more options available, depending on whether the person one is confronting is a colleague, a superior, or a subordinate in the organization. If, in fact, the first four steps have not worked in a confrontational setting and the behavior is still unacceptable and must be confronted, then the supervisor has one of two choices, depending on the relationship.

If confronting a person at the same or at a higher level in the organization, the next step would be to make a *formal request*. A formal request should contain information from each of the four previously described elements—namely, a description of the problem, expression of the effect the problem is creating, specification of alternative ways to act, and some elaboration on the consequences of those alternatives. The formal request should be in writing and it should be conveyed in a formal manner.

If the supervisor is confronting someone who reports to him or her in the chain of command, then the next step is to give a *direct order*. Again, the direct order at this stage of the process should be in writing, it should contain the same elements that were previously communicated verbally, and it should be passed on to the person in a formal setting. The setting at this stage of the game will usually be a disciplinary type of meeting and probably is the step at the disciplinary process at which written reprimand is being used so the direct order would be in the form of a written reprimand.

If, in fact, the direct order with a direct request does not work, then the supervisor may be confronting a situation in which a communication breakdown has occurred. If the breakdown is with someone in the organization to whom the supervisor reports, then the supervisor should seriously consider looking elsewhere for employment. If the breakdown is with someone who reports to the supervisor, then the supervisor should make it clear to that person that the probability for a continued, productive working relationship is minimal, and that termination may result in the near future.

Not all supervisory situations are this challenging or this difficult, but some are challenging in a different way. In one challenging and unusual situation, for example, the supervisor is required to make a formal presentation. (This problem will be discussed in the next section.)

Giving Presentations

As health care organizations become larger and more complex, we are forced to rely on more formal means for the transmission of relevant information. Presentations are required in staff meetings, in-service sessions, committee meetings, board meetings, and patient education programs. Whatever the setting, several basic steps are beneficial in helping one to prepare for the formal presentation, and a number of guidelines are useful in making the delivery. Morrisey (1968), for example, identified a six-step process for preparing to deliver a formal presentation.

Step 1.   Establish objectives and identify a reason for the presentation. Why is it being given? What outcomes are hoped for? Will people be expected to act differently as a result of having attended this presentation? If so, how do I characterize that action?

Step 2.   Analyze your audience. Who will be attending? What are their primary needs? What do they hope to gain from the presentation? What is the best information processing mode for them to operate within? How do they usually process information? What will make this information comfortable for them? Will you be saying anything that conflicts directly with any of their needs? What are their most pressing concerns relative to the content of your presentation?

Step 3.   Prepare a preliminary plan for the presentation. The preliminary plan should identify the specific objectives for the briefing, the specific audience for whom the presentation is intended, and the main ideas or concepts that the audience must understand for the objectives to be met. It should also identify the type of information needed to back up the points that will be made in the presentation. The plan should be used as a guide for both the briefer in selecting the proper materials and during final presentation preparation and for other people who may be involved either in setting up the presentation or in ensuring that it is successful.

Step 4.   Select resource material for the presentation. Nothing is more disappointing than to hear a presenter state points that cannot be backed up with facts or supporting evidence. Powerful presenters ensure that that have adequate evidence to convince the audience of the validity of their information. Presenters without supportive material and without facts appear amateurish and have less impact.

Step 5.   Organize the material for the most effective presentation possible. The organization should include an introduction, a body or substance section, and a closing or conclusion. An example of an effective format might be, first, to provide a direct statement of an introduction outlining the purpose and objectives for the presentation. Second, develop the ideas and present the information people should understand adequately and, third, conclude with a review of purpose and appeal for action and a compelling summary of the information that was presented.

Step 6.   Practice the presentation in advance. A number of techniques can be used to accomplish this objective. You might give the presentation to yourself in front of a mirror. Practice aloud. Ideas always sound differently when voiced aloud than when they are written on paper. There is no substitute for hearing your ideas prior to appearing in front of the audience. You might use a tape recorder. This can also be beneficial because you can hear what you have said after you have said it. A final way to practice is to stage an actual practice presentation in front of co-workers or colleagues. There is no substitute for practice. The more important the presentation, the more important it is to practice the presentation so that it runs smoothly.

In delivering the actual presentation, effective presenters might also do the following:

1. Be sincere
2. Be cheerful and friendly
3. Pause for a moment before starting
4. Talk to your audience
5. Maintain eye contact with members of the audience
6. Use natural gestures to emphasize points
7. Personalize you talk by referring to members of the audience as you talk
8. Use video aids
9. Use simple language and short sentences
10. Drive home your points with relevant stories
11. Avoid trite or stale expressions
12. Quit while you still have audience interest

In contrast to these guidelines, actions that experienced presenters have learned to avoid include the following:

1. Do not apologize
2. Do not exaggerate
3. Do not lean or slouch over the lectern
4. Do not smoke or chew gum
5. Do not conspicuously look at your watch
6. Do not run your sentences together with ''and''
7. Do not pass out literature until your presentation is finished
8. Do not use other repetitive phrases or words

Few things can provide more excitement and a greater feeling of accomplishment than the delivery of an effective presentation. Almost everyone is nervous and anxious prior to making an important presentation. It is helpful to use this anxiety and tension to create a more dynamic and forceful presentation. When making a presentation, concentrate on your strengths. Do the things that you do well. Avoid placing yourself in a situation in which you are relying on certain skills or abilities with which you are personally not comfortable. Humor is an area in which people experience trouble. Humor can be valuable in a presentation in several ways. A point can be made with humor that cannot be made as effectively any other way. Humor can also be a tension reliever. Tension builds in a group when someone makes a wisecrack; after the laughter subsides, the tension often dissipates. Humor can also be used to establish a bond with the audience. But it can do this only if the humor is tasteful and is not used at someone else's expense. Ethnic, racist, or gender-specific humor have no place in the communications of an effective supervisor.

One final area of communication important to the supervisor is that of written correspondence.

Corresponding in Writing

Written communication is as important for health care supervisors as face-to-face verbal communication. The correspondence generated by health care supervisors becomes an important source of historical data that can affect how a particular case might be handled. A supervisor's letter might also be crucial in determining whether a specific policy is adopted. Many important decisions can be affected by the quality of information contained in a supervisor's letter, memorandum, or report. It is even possible that a supervisor's written correspondence might sometime become a critical piece of evidence in a legal proceeding. Thus it is important that written correspondence be prepared with care.

Our emphasis here will not be on the grammatical aspects of good writing. It is assumed that supervisors can learn the techniques of correct grammar elsewhere. Numerous books exist to accomplish this goal. Rather, the focus here is on the structural elements that are most critical to a supervisor's effectiveness in using the written word. The following guidelines will help health care supervisors to achieve power in their written correspondence.

Limit Each Document to One Objective for a Single Purpose.   If the document is a letter, ask yourself: "What do I want the reader to do as a result of reading this letter?" If it's a written memorandum, you might ask: "How do I want people to respond to this memo?" If you have more than one objective or multiple purposes, it is usually best to use multiple documents, that is, one for each purpose.

State Your Purpose at the Beginning.   Tell the reader what you want in the first sentence. Give your reasons later. Structure your correspondence the way journalists structure newspaper articles. Position the most important information at the beginning so that if someone stops reading, he or she will have missed the least important information.

Write the Same Way You Talk.   Use active verbs. Avoid trite and formal expressions. For example, instead of saying, "Your attention is requested in the following matter . . .," say: "I'd like you to know." Avoid using words or phrases that sound arrogant or pompous. Write simply and in a straightforward manner.

Use Appropriate References to Individuals.   Use personal pronouns and individual names. When talking about people, make sure that you refer to the person with whatever form is most natural.

Consistently Use Short, Simple Words.   Approximately three-fourths of the time you should use words that are one syllable long. Multisyllable words make reading more difficult and are often misunderstood. The simplest word that conveys the appropriate meaning is the best.

Use Short Sentences.   An average sentence in your writing should contain no more than seventeen words. Longer sentences detract from the meaning and lessen the impact. Effective writers work hard to create powerful, easily understood sentences.

Keep Paragraphs Short.   Paragraphs of three to five sentences are adequate for most written communication. Paragraphs help the reader process the information and retain the information more effectively. Again, write like the journalist. Keep words and sentences short and simple and join them together in paragraphs that convey precise thoughts.

Limit the Length of the Entire Document.   Most letters and certainly most memorandums can achieve their objectives in less than one page. If much of your correspondence is longer than a single page, you are probably saying too much. Your effectiveness will diminish correspondingly.

Include a Strong Ending.   A powerful conclusion is important for effective written communication. This might be a statement of a deadline, an appeal for action, or a request for confirmation that the message has been received. Whatever is appropriate based on the objective of the specific document being constructed, it is important that the ending be strong.

Make Sure Your Written Communication Looks Attractive.   Written correspondence represents you in your absence. Take pride in the image you project. Leave adequate margins, indent paragraphs properly, use short paragraphs, and use attractive type styles and good quality paper.

Send Copies Only to Those Who Need Them.   Do not send a copy to a recipient's superior unless it is a letter of praise. If there is doubt regarding whether a person should receive a copy, do not send that person a copy. It is probably unnecessary.

In summary, the best advice regarding written communication is to be precise and concise. Do not generate any more paperwork than is necessary. When it is necessary, however, make sure it counts.

Receiving Skills

Communication is often viewed as a means of influence. This is especially true when it is addressed in the context of supervision. Most typically, the emphasis is on directing, persuading, or confronting. All three of these concepts are important. However, receiving is as important as sending to a supervisor. Receivers can have as much impact on the communication process as senders.

We rarely think of the listener as being the influencer in the communication process; however, the way in which a receiver listens can have even greater impact on the efficiency of the process than what the sender does. This impact is crucial to a supervisor's overall success. Good supervisors are good listeners.

Like most supervisory traits, good listening skills can be developed. Practice the following and your effectiveness as a communicater and as a supervisor will improve significantly.

Be Sincerely Interested in What the Sender Has To Say.   Notice the choice of words here. The message does not say ''act'' interested nor does it say pretend or feign interest. The message is clear: Be interested. If you, as a supervisor, are not interested in most of what people have to say, then you should seriously consider whether you are in the right position. If your job is important to you, it should not be difficult to maintain a sincere interest most of the time in what people have to say.

Judge Content Not Delivery.   Do not be a poor listener because the sender lacks strong sending skills. In most situations, people can learn and can practice good interpersonal communication skills. Many people, however, do not know how to communicate in ways that are likely to satisfy their needs in the most efficient manner. Even if someone is not a good sender, do not allow yourself to be a poor communicator.

Don't Get "Hooked" into Emotional Responses.   Hold your fire. Be calm. Collect your thoughts before responding. Try to hear beyond the emotionally loaded messages that are being sent to discover the sender's real needs and true feelings. Then carefully respond in a way that encourages those needs to be handled in a straightforward and direct manner.

Listen for Ideas.   Keep a ''big picture'' perspective. Many times people have major ideas or concepts behind the messages they are transmitting verbally. When those messages are transmitted, however, we often hear the verbal bits and pieces and sometimes fail to tie everything together in a comprehensive way that leads to better understanding. Seek this understanding. Tie ideas together. Search for themes and concepts.

Be Flexible.   The best communicators often adapt their style to match the style of the person they are communicating with. Pace yourself to match the rhythm and the mood of the sender. Be willing to handle issues at a pace that is comfortable for the sender. Be responsive to the content in the sender's message. Do not lock yourself into first impressions. Allow yourself flexibility as greater understanding is achieved.

Work at Being a Good Listener.   Concentrate on using good listening skills. Haphazard listeners are poor listeners. Practice all the time and consistently try to improve. Good listeners make a conscious effort to apply the best listening techniques when they are in the receiving mode.

Resist Distraction. Control the environment. Avoid interruptions. Pay attention. If the telephone rings, politely tell the caller you are involved in a meeting and ask him or her to call back later. Close the door if necessary or move to another setting. Most important, take charge so that you can concentrate on listening.

Exercise Your Mind. Maintain mental flexibility. The more nimble your mind is, the better you will listen.

Keep an Open Mind. The worst assumption a supervisor can make is that he or she knows it all. To the contrary, assume that you do not know it all. Have confidence in what you are doing but operate on the assumption that there is a better way to do it somewhere and it is your responsibility to do it. The only way you will do it is through effective listening. There is something to learn from everyone. Make it a goal to learn what you can from each person you communicate with.

Capitalize on Your Thinking Speed. Listeners have a distinct advantage over senders because they think at a rate that is four to five times faster than the rate at which a speaker speaks. Use this thinking speed to analyze the content of the sender's message, to evaluate nonverbal signals that are being sent, to determine meaning and underlying needs of the sender, and to use power constructively in your listening processes (Sigband, 1969).

All these guidelines point the listener in a specific direction. That direction is intended to make the sender feel important and worthwhile. The better the sender feels about what he or she has to say, the more effective the communication process will be. It is the listener's responsibility to provide this feeling of worthwhileness and self-respect.

Whether sending or receiving, however, the supervisor is responsible for maintaining an organizational environment that enhances constructive communication processes on an ongoing basis. Some principles for achieving this goal are presented in the next section.

MAINTAINING A HEALTHY COMMUNICATION ENVIRONMENT

A supervisor can use different techniques to maintain a healthy communication environment. Maintaining good planning habits, especially through using some of the methods of managing by objectives discussed in earlier chapters, contributes to a healthy environment. Organizing properly and setting standards for performance and communicating those standards also help. Applying effective leadership techniques and good management practices will make a significant difference. Good supervisory practices will help to maintain an environment in which good communication habits will develop and flourish.

The American Management Association (AMA) developed a number of communication principles that specifically defined what supervisors and managers can do to maintain a healthy organizational environment. These guidelines were called The Ten Commandments of Good Communication and were designed to improve the effectiveness of organizational communication. Summarized briefly they are as follows (AMA, 1955):

1. *Seek to calrify your ideas before communicating.* The more systematically we analyze the problem or idea to be communicated, the clearer it becomes. Good planning must consider the goals and attitudes of those who will receive the communication and those who will be affected by it.

2. *Examine the true purpose of each communication.* Before you communicate, ask yourself what you *really* want to accomplish with your message. Do you want to obtain information, initiate action, change another person's attitude? Identify your most important goal and then adapt your language, time, and total approach to serve that specific objective.

3. *Consider the total physical and human setting whenever you communicate.* Meaning and intent are conveyed by more than words alone. Consider, for example, your sense of timing, the circumstances under which you make an announcement or render a decision, and the physical setting, as well as the social climate, customs, and past practices of your organization.

4. *Consult with others where appropriate in planning communication.* Consultation often helps to lend additional insight and objectivity to your message. Moreover, those who have helped you plan your communication will give it their active support.

5. *Consider while you communicate the overtones as well as the basic content of your message.* Your tone of voice, your expression, your apparent receptiveness to the responses of others—all have tremendous impact on those you wish to reach. Frequently overlooked, these subtleties of communication often affect a listener's reaction to a message even more than its basic content will.

6. *Take the opportunity when it arises to convey something of help or value to the receiver.* Consideration of the other person's interests and needs—the habit of trying to look at things from the other person's point of view—will frequently reveal opportunities to convey something of immediate benefit for a long-range value to the other person.

7. *Follow up your communication.* Do this by asking questions, by encouraging the receiver to express reactions, by follow-up contacts, or by subsequent review of performance. Make sure that every important communication includes a feedback process so that complete understanding and appropriate action can be tested.

8. *Communicate for tomorrow as well as today.* Communications may be aimed primarily at meeting the demands of an immediate situation. They must be planned with the past in mind if they are to maintain consistency in the receiver's view. But most important, they must be consistent with long-range interests and goals. To this extent, future effects must be considered as well. For example, it is not easy to communicate frankly on such matters as performance of a subordinate, but postponing disagreeable communication

makes it only more difficult in the long run and is actually unfair to the people involved.

9. *Be sure your actions support your communications.* The most persuasive kind of communication is not what you say but what you do. For every supervisor, this statement means that good supervisory practices—such as clear assignment of responsibility and authority, fair rewards for effort, and sound policy enforcement—serve to communicate more effectively than all the gifts of oratory.

10. *Seek not only to be understood but also to understand—be a good listener.* When we start talking, we often cease to listen. Listening demands that we concentrate not only on the explicit meanings another person is expressing, but also on the implicit meanings, unspoken words, and undertones that may be far more significant.

SUMMARY

Nothing in organizations can be accomplished without effective communication. Communication involves sending and receiving. However, a supervisor's responsibility for effective communications transcends simply having the skills to talk or to listen. The supervisor must also ensure that his or her actions create an ongoing environment in which effective communications can occur and that everyone in the organization communicates to the best of his or her ability in ways that allow his or her needs and the needs of the organization to be met consistently and on an ongoing basis.

REFERENCES

American Management Associations. *Ten Commandments of Good Communication.* Chicago: American Management Association, 1955.

Bower, S. A., & Bower, G. H. *Asserting Yourself.* Reading, MA: Addison-Wesley, 1976.

Gordon, T. *P.E.T. (Parent Effectiveness Training).* New York: Wyden, 1970.

Haney, W. V. *Communication and Organizational Behavior* (3rd ed.). Homewood, IL: Irwin, 1973.

Morrisey, G. L. *Effective Business and Technical Presentations.* Reading, MA: Addison-Wesley, 1968.

Sigband, N. B. *Communication for Management.* Glenview, IL: Scott, Foresman, 1969.

Chapter Seven

Problem Solving and Decision Making

In a recent continuing education course for nurses in supervisory positions, one student stated: "If only I could find some way to get rid of all the problems I have to deal with every day, then I wouldn't have any trouble at all supervising my floor the way it should be supervised." This is similar to a remark another student made a few years ago: "I don't mind supervising. In fact I think supervising is both enjoyable and rewarding. What I don't like to do is make decisions—now *that's* something I could definitely do without."

Both of these comments are somewhat naive because supervisors will always be confronted with problems to solve and decisions to make. As long as it takes people to perform the work in organizations, and as long as the work they provide is complex and important, problems are inevitable and decisions will be commonplace. Thus the supervisor who wants to be effective in total job performance must learn how to solve problems and to make decisions.

Management theorists once believed and taught that problems and conflicts in organizations were both unnecessary and harmful. These people thought that the presence of either problems or conflicts in an organization indicated that something was seriously wrong. The belief was that problems arose only if the supervisors and managers in the organization were doing something wrong. In general, *this attitude* is now viewed as incorrect for several reasons. First, problems in organizations are inevitable. Problems will naturally arise while one is fulfilling the purposes of the organization—any organization. It does not seem productive to view something that is inevitable and natural as wrong. Second, the adoption of such an attitude encourages people to either overlook or avoid problems that legitimately arise.

Imagine yourself telling a patient with the flu or a cold that something is basically wrong with him or her as a person merely because he or she happens to be afflicted with something undesirable at the moment. Such a statement would be ridiculous. Instead, you would probably think about that person in the following terms: "Well, here's a person that is probably as good as any other, but temporarily is not performing as well as usual because of this minor illness. The sooner we treat it, the sooner this person will return to a normal level of functioning.'' Then you would do your part to see that a thorough diagnosis is completed and the best possible course of action is developed to restore the person to the healthiest possible condition. This is the same type of attitude that should be adopted in handling supervisory problems. Similar to the patient who is ill, if the problems are ignored, they only become worse. The most effective way to achieve healthy, efficient organizational practices is to recognize that problems will arise, anticipate what they might be before they surface, and confront them objectively in the best possible way when they occur.

Similar to problem solving, decision making is also a key part of every supervisor's role, and the two are interrelated. Supervisors must not only make decisions for themselves, but must also make them for others. When to schedule breaks, how to organize work, what to do about employees who violate some of the rules of the organization, which concerns should be given the highest priority or the most emphasis, are only a few of the endless series of decisions a supervisor is expected to make daily. The better a supervisor's ability to make decisions, the more satisfaction he or she will gain from doing the job. To help improve both decision-making and problem-solving abilities, this chapter will first present a definition of both problems and decisions and will then discuss the different types of problems and decisions a health care supervisor might encounter. Finally, a method for solving problems and making decisions that has been valuable for thousands of other supervisors will be described.

WHAT IS A PROBLEM?

If you want to cause someone to become perplexed in a rather short period of time, ask him or her what a problem is. Do not settle for an example of a problem, but ask the person to define the word problem for you. Stop for a moment and think. What is a problem? Can you define the term?

When asked this question, most people respond by stating: ''A problem is something that needs an answer.'' Or: ''Something that needs a solution.'' Although both may be true statements regarding problems, neither is close to defining the term. Since it has been our experience that a sound understanding of what problems are substantially helps in solving them, we will start with defining a problem.

Problems are obstacles, conditions, or phenomena that either: (1) stand in the way of achieving objectives or (2) cause a deviation from the desired status. In both cases, problems are undesirable factors that must be handled if the desired results of the organization are to be achieved. These factors (obstacles, conditions, or phenomena) can be human, operational, or technical in nature. Because of the undesirability of these factors, they must be resolved somehow. They could be either eliminated or circumnavigated; at the least, their adverse effects must be eliminated or neutralized. Consider the following examples.

Assume you work in a small clinic in which much of the routine laboratory work is accomplished on the premises. On a particularly busy day, numerous blood samples are taken for routine analysis. While preparing to conduct the intended lab work, you discover that the centrifuge is not working properly. Because of this breakdown, you cannot complete the lab work as intended. This would be an example of the first type of problem—one in which obstacles, conditions, or phenomena stand in the way of achieving objectives. In this case, your objective is to conduct a routine analysis and the breakdown of equipment prevents you from doing so.

Now place yourself in the same clinic with the following different set of circumstances. Assume that you have general supervisory responsibilities for the entire clinic, including the responsibilities for the financial operations. For some time you have been overseeing this operation by reviewing monthly cash flow statements and a balance sheet prepared by the person who handles all the billings. One day it occurs to you that the flow of money seems to be a bit sluggish and not quite what you would have expected based on the operating level of the clinic during this time. With the person who is handling these matters, you begin to review the situation. While reviewing individual files, you discover that some of the patients are behind in payment of their bills. Further investigation reveals a serious accounts receivable problem, with tens of thousands of dollars more than 30 days past due. This type of problem differs from the first one presented because the circumstances describe *a deviation* from the desired level or standard of performance rather than *an obstacle* standing in the way of achieving objectives. Both problems, however, are serious and must be resolved. The responsibility for handling them is the supervisor's.

With the exception of certain types of mechanical failure or equipment breakdown, no two problems are the same. Rarely, if ever, is a supervisor likely to encounter two problems that are identical. Contrary to the popular myth, history never repeats itself exactly.

However, different categories of problems often contain similar characteristics. Understanding of these categories and the commonalities of the problems within each category can be helpful to a manager.

Different Categories of Problems

Three fundamental categories of problems, grouped together because of the types of variables they include are (1) people, (2) operational, and (3) technical.

People Problems.   This category includes all the problems of supervision that are caused primarily by the actions or behavior of a specific individual or group of people. These are problems in which the solutions will be arrived at by causing behavioral changes. Consider the following examples.

> Jane L. has worked as a ward clerk at Community Hospital for about a year and a half. She works well with others and is an outstanding employee in every regard except that she arrives at work a minimum of 10 minutes late every day without fail. She shows concern for her tardiness by working the discrepant time into her

lunch period. Although her fellow employees are aware of her make-up time, they feel she is receiving special treatment from the supervisor and resent her continued tardiness. Although the supervisor has tried various methods with Jane to correct the situation, the tardiness continues. The other workers are complaining and a noticeable decline in work performance is occurring.

Mary W. is a laboratory technician at Spritz Memorial Hospital. She has worked there for twelve years and is a good worker. She carries out any task and does her work according to all the procedures and regulations. She can repeat verbatim any regulation concerning work or union rules. The problem is that she is disruptive with fellow employees. She spreads rumors, exaggerates minor conflicts, and constantly tries to show higher levels of the hospital administration in a bad light. All her co-workers dislike and distrust her. Morale is becoming worse all the time.

The key to solving people problems is generally to cause people to change their behavior. Sometimes the best approach is through confrontation. But behavioral changes often result from policy changes or rule modifications as well. The important factor to remember, however, is the focus on behavior.

Operational Problems. Some problems are caused primarily by factors other than people or technology. They include such things as policy, organizational structure, dynamics of the marketplace or the economy, and problems stemming from laws and regulations. Operational problems differ from people problems in that they are usually more tangible, making it easier for the problem solver to isolate and analyze the variables in the problem. Whereas human behavior often seems vague and the causes of people problems seem ambiguous, the substance of operational problems is usually more concrete. Operational problems are not by nature more or less challenging, nor are they by nature more or less important than people problems. However, they are different.

The problem regarding delinquent receivables mentioned earlier in this chapter is an example of an operational problem. It falls into this category because the source of the problem's cause is systemic in nature rather than human or technical. The problem exists because of the lack of an effective and workable procedure for handling accounts receivable. No matter who might be requested to work in the receivables position, the problem would exist—it is not unique to a particular person. The solution lies in developing a method to make certain the accounts are always under control, regardless of who is performing the clerical work.

Technical Problems. Some problems are caused primarily by mechanical, technical, electrical, electronic, or hydraulic equipment component and/or system functioning or failure to function. Although many technical problems are extremely difficult and challenging to solve, the category of technical problems is probably the easiest to understand. The example mentioned earlier regarding the breakdown of the laboratory centrifuge is one example of a technical problem.

The health field is somewhat unique compared to other fields and to industry in that supervisors other than maintenance or engineering supervisors are usually *not* expected to solve technical problems. Expert technicians are usually called on to solve technical problems.

With these ideas regarding problems in mind, let us turn to the topic of decisions.

WHAT IS A DECISION?

Most simply stated, a decision is a choice among alternatives. Supervisors make a wide variety of decisions constantly. Decisions may include such routine matters as deciding on the brand of products to be used in different areas or who should work on which shifts and when employees will be allowed time off for vacations. They may also include more complex choices, such as whether to add a new wing to the floor, or whether new types of services should be added to those already being offered. Whether routine or unique, minor or major, it is the supervisor who must decide—or at least prepare others to decide—what action should be taken. The supervisor decides and others carry out the actions determined by the choice.

The nature of different decisions varies considerably. Because of changing circumstances, no two decisions are ever likely to be the same. However, that does *not* mean that different decisions cannot be approached in a similar manner. In fact, several factors are commonly found in all decisions and problems.

In the following sections, we will examine some of the issues relevant to deciding who should be assigned the responsibility for solving different problems and making decisions, and we will discuss a methods to use when you are the problem solver or decision maker.

WHO SHOULD BE ASSIGNED TO THE TASK?

The first question a supervisor should ask when confronted with a problem or decision is: "Should I or should I not assume responsibility for responding to this issue?" There is a tendency among supervisors to rush off immediately to confront every concern that is expressed regardless of the merits or potential benefit to be derived from such a confrontation. The most practical way to develop this habit of consciously deciding whether to act is to ask yourself the following three questions any time a new decision or problem arises.

1. What would happen if I ignored this?
2. Is action warranted?
3. Is now the best time to confront this issue?

Only if the answers to these questions indicate a strong positive conclusion that action is warranted should the supervisor proceed with problem-solving or decision-making activity. After the supervisor has decided that the issue is under his or her area of responsibility, the next concern should be whom to assign the work to.

Results quite frequently depend as much on who does the work as on any other factor. Yet quite often, supervisors arbitrarily select those to be involved in different decision-making and problem-solving activities. In most cases, this tendency results from habit. For example, some supervisors prefer to keep things fairly confidential. Consequently, they do most of this work themselves without soliciting much input or participation from others. On the other hand, some supervisors prefer to involve as many people as possible in as many different activities as possible. In each case, the supervisor is probably following the *most comfortable* course of action, one that has evolved for several years and is now followed from habit. The only drawback is that, although the supervisor will be most comfortable always doing things basically the same, the results will be inferior. The same approach simply cannot be the best strategy for every circumstance. *Comfort does not equate to best.* The following choices exist for involving different people in decision-making and problem-solving activities:

1. Assign the responsibility to the most qualified person.
2. Assign the responsibility to any qualified person.
3. Do it yourself.
4. Assign it simultaneously to two or more people who will act independently.
5. Divide the assignment, giving different parts to different people.
6. Assign it to a group who will work together.
7. Hire a consultant—ask an expert.
8. Delegate to whomever has the most available time.
9. Assign to people who most need the experience.
10. Two or more of the above.

In deciding who should be involved in the process, the following factors should be considered:

1. Technical or special knowledge requirements necessary to resolve the issue.
2. Experience requirements necessary to understand the situation completely.
3. The need for skills in the area of problem solving or decision making.
4. Who will be affected by the outcome.
5. Who has something at stake (to either gain or lose) in the outcome.
6. The need for credibility in the process.
7. The overall mix of both quality and acceptance of final solution.
8. The need for backup alternatives.
9. The need for diversity in different approaches.
10. The need to minimize possible adverse personal consequences.
11. Political requirements (both internal and external to the organization).
12. Who can benefit most from this assignment.

These factors should be considered for every new problem or decision of any significance. The relative level of importance will vary with each new set of circumstances. Another way to consider the most important dimensions is to develop the habit of asking the following four questions before taking on any problem or decision:

1. Who should be involved in the process?
2. Who should be consulted before the final decision?
3. Who should be informed afterwards?
4. Who should be responsible for managing the process?

Failure to consider any of these factors before beginning the actual work of solving problems or making decisions will invariably make the process more cumbersome and time-consuming in the long run, and results will suffer accordingly. After considering these factors, one starts the actual work of problem solving and decision making. The following method will increase the probability of achieving top-notch results in this area.

HOW TO SOLVE PROBLEMS AND MAKE DECISIONS

Although many different approaches are taught for solving problems and making decisions, a supervisor in the health field will probably obtain the best results by learning to use the *Lyles Method*. This simple, straightforward technique was devised by one of the authors for everyday use by managers and supervisors (Lyles, 1982). This method is advantageous for the supervisor because it is both practical and results-oriented, without being cumbersome or difficult to manage.

As shown in Figure 7.1, the Lyles Method consists of six steps when applied to decision making and seven steps when applied to problem solving. Only the last six steps are used when making decisions, as indicated by the arrows on the left. When problems are encountered, however, all seven steps are used, as indicated by the arrows on the right.

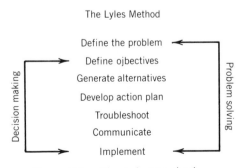

Figure 7.1.   The Lyles' Method.

A major difference between this method and most others is its focus on achieving the desired final results. This is specifically demonstrated in the second, fifth, and sixth steps of the problem-solving process. Because defining objectives, troubleshooting, and communication are activities that make an important difference between finding the right answer and finally achieving the desired results, they add to the effectiveness of the problem-solving or decision-making process. Combined with the other four steps, these three factors provide a powerful, yet practical approach that is described in detail as follows.

Step 1: Define the Problem.

When confronted with a problem, start by defining it. To define the problem, *identify* and *describe* the obstacles, conditions, or phenomena that either (1) stand in the way of achieving objectives or (2) cause a deviation from the desired status. Problems exist when something is wrong. A problem is well defined when the supervisor understands it sufficiently so that he or she can explain the situation to others in terms they will understand *and* can generate possible solutions that will eliminate the problem.

When a problem arises, a supervisor is already in the process of doing something—of trying to achieve results. A problem is a problem only if it interferes with

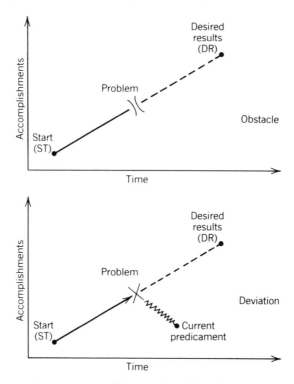

Figure 7.2. Problem as obstacle or deviation.

| FORMAT #1: | (A very specific causal condition, event, or phenomenon), **IS PREVENTING** (very specific **desired** results), **FROM HAPPENING.** |
| FORMAT #2: | (A very specific causal condition, event, or phenomenon), **IS CAUSING** (very specific **undesired** results) **TO OCCUR.** |

Figure 7.3. Format for defining problems.

attempts to accomplish these results in some significant way. Either it stands in the way (obstacle) or it causes some other, undesired result to occur (deviation). If, for example, the supervisor is trying to move from point A to point B, the effects of the problem could be illustrated as shown in Figure 7.2 below. To define the problem adequately, therefore, a supervisor must be able to specify the following: achieve desired end results (DR) originally intended; how the problem conditions interfere with the attainment of these results; and what actually caused the interference.

When defining problems, it is helpful to remember a specific format for the problem definition. This step is necessary not because the process or method for solving a problem is more important than the results, but because it simply helps the problem solver to think through the most important factors surrounding the problem and to keep them in their proper perspective. Depending on the type of problem, you could use either one of the two formats shown in Figure 7.3 to state the definition of a problem.

The first format is used to define problems in the form of obstacles, and the second is used to define problems in the form of deviations. Only after a problem definition that fits one of these formats has been established should the problem solver proceed to the second step of the process.

Step 2: Define Objectives

Although this is the second step in the method, as well as the second step in problem solving, *define objectives* is the first step to be used when making decisions.

The supervisor's objectives and the goals of the entire organization should not change with every passing problem or decision. However, it is important that supervisors know exactly how the solution to every problem and the result of each decision relates to the organization's ongoing objectives. Every action the supervisor takes should be compatible with the overall scheme of operations.

When solving problems and making decisions, define objectives on two levels. First, the supervisor should make certain the overall objectives in this area of responsibility are understood and specified. Second, the objectives of the particular management action being considered should be clearly defined. The following guidelines will help to define objectives when you are solving problems and making decisions.

1. If there is a problem involved, make sure it is completely understood before attempting to formulate objectives.
2. Set objectives that focus on results and intended outcomes. Stay away from the "how to." (Methods for accomplishing objectives will be developed in the third step of the process, *generate alternatives.*)
3. Assume that not everything is known, that new opportunities are waiting to be discovered, and that your opinions are probably obsolete.
4. Question everything; do not take anything for granted.
5. Do not waste time setting objectives for things that will happen anyway.
6. Be specific. Focus as much as possible on *measurable* factors, *tangible* end results, and *quantifiable* outcomes.
7. Make sure your objectives are feasible.
8. Be reasonably consistent. This is *not* to say you should be rigid and inflexible. However, a certain amount of consistency is important.

Objectives specify the end-result outcomes you desire to accomplish. They tell us where you want to end up. Alternative courses of action are different ways to accomplish goals. Thus generating alternatives is the next step of the process.

Step 3: Generate Alternatives

Generating alternatives involves more than merely contemplating things to do. It also involves developing specific courses of action that will lead to the accomplishment of previously defined objectives.

The most practical method for generating alternatives for the kinds of problems health care supervisors encounter is through brainstorming. Although brainstorming can be done by an individual, the best results are usually achieved when the activities are carried out by a small group of ten people or less. The process itself is quite simple.

The group meets and first spends a reasonable amount of time ensuring that each group member fully understands the objectives of the decision and has a common vision regarding the desired end results. If they are working to solve a problem, everyone should understand the problem completely. The members then begin thinking of alternative ways to accomplish the objectives. As the alternatives are generated, one or two members of the group record them (on a chalkboard or flip chart where all can see them) as quickly as possible *as stated* by the originator. The process should be intense and uninhibited, with everyone trying to develop as many new and different ideas as possible. Discussion or evaluation of individual ideas should be avoided at this time because it will tend to slow down the process and dampen enthusiasm and creativity.

The following ground rules are suggested for brainstorming sessions. They will be most effective when written out on flip chart paper or posterboard and posted in the meeting room. They should be reviewed at the start of the session and referred to whenever someone violates one or more of them.

1. Everyone tries their best to develop as many new and different alternatives as possible.
2. Anything is acceptable. No ''bad'' ideas exist. Evaluation will start later.
3. Do not evaluate, criticize, or discuss any ideas during the brainstorming process.
4. Generate as many different alternatives as possible.
5. Use the ideas of others to stimulate your own thinking. Try to improve on them or combine them to suggest better approaches.
6. Encourage each other. Work as a group to develop a group product, rather than entering into competition with each other.

The most common problem in brainstroming is that brainstormers frequently are trapped by their previous experiences. This causes the brainstorming session to be more of a memory testing exercise than an exercise in creativity. Recalling old techniques is not necessarily bad, but if it is the only source of ideas for the group, the results will suffer. Brainstorming is most effective when it fosters creativity and the development of *new and different* ideas.

Once a healthy list of alternatives has been developed, it is then appropriate to proceed with the next step in the process, which is to develop a course of action.

Step 4: Develop Action Plan

Now is the time to analyze and compare the different courses of action proposed, and to select one. First, choose the course of action that is best for the circumstances. The following *ten commandments for choosing a course of action* will help facilitate this process.

1. Focus on the total end result to be achieved.
2. Never accept your final choice as being final.
3. At least 80 percent of the time, choose an alternative other than the first one considered—you can almost always do better.
4. Do not do anything solely because it worked once before. Choose actions that are clearly justified based on the demands of the current situation.
5. Never follow the advice of experts unless the advice makes complete sense to you.
6. Always trust your own intuition. A hunch is a conclusion based on facts you previously observed and stored.
7. Remember that after you act, things will change. Always be prepared to handle new circumstances and to respond to new information.
8. Be bold rather than timid. Major changes are easier to implement and more likely to take hold than minor changes.
9. Assess the needs and priorities of other people and design an action plan that is supportive of them.

ACTION PLAN

Objectives: _____

_____

_____

_____

Specific Actions	Who	Cost	By When

Figure 7.4.   Format for action plan.

10. Take enough time to decide. Haste does tend to make waste (particularly in management decisions), so do not rush things.

Although these factors will not guarantee success in every case, if you use them and remain sensitive to the issues they raise, you will most certainly improve the overall quality of the action plans you develop.

After chosing a basic course of action, you will develop a more formal plan of action. In the plan, it is important to specify time, cost factors, objectives, end results, and accountability. The form presented in Figure 7.4 is a simple way to summarize this information.

If you can complete this action planning form with reasonable specificity, you should have a fairly detailed idea of what to do. However, before trying to implement the plan, two additional steps should be taken. The first step is to troubleshoot.

Step 5: Troubleshoot

The most efficient problem solving possible is problem solving in advance—in essence, "solving" problems before they become problems. This means taking care of potential problems (or their causes) before they can interfere with your intended actions.

Troubleshooting means to conduct a critical review of the action plan for potential problems or additional benefits that might result from the implementation of the plan. A simple yet thorough way to conduct a troubleshooting review is to ask the following questions about your plan:

1. Are the objectives of the plan sound, desirable, and understood?
2. What is the likelihood (or probability) the proposed course of action will achieve the objectives?
3. Are staffing plans adequate to fulfill the action?
4. Have plans been made to capitalize on collateral advantages? (What other benefits must be accrued from the implementation of this plan?)
5. Is the plan to communicate sufficiently detailed so that support will be generated and all those affected will know what to expect?
6. What are the disadvantages of the proposed action?
7. In what ways can the course of action fail?
8. Who might want to see it fail?
9. Is the proposed course of action likely to embarrass anyone, such as top management, the medical staff, another department, or the patients?
10. Why do anything at all? Why do this?
11. Is the time frame realistic and feasible?
12. Is there a better time to act?
13. Are there special conditions that may have been overlooked that could throw this plan off schedule?
14. Why do it this way? Can you think of a better way?
15. Who else should give approval or be informed of the decision?
16. Is the course of action truly cost effective? If you were spending your own money, is this how you would spend it?
17. Does anything about the proposed course of action make you feel at all uneasy or uncomfortable?

If these questions are asked routinely for all plans that you as a supervisor are asked to review and approve, you will probably eliminate between 25 percent and 40 percent of the problems you would otherwise encounter.

Perhaps one of the more powerful examples of effective troubleshooting is described in the following situation:

A new hospital administrator, holding his first staff meeting, thought that a rather difficult matter had been settled to everyone's satisfaction, when one of the participants suddenly asked: "Would this have satisfied Nurse Bryan?" At once the argument started all over and did not subside until a new and much more ambitious solution to the problem had been hammered out.

Nurse Bryan, the administrator learned, had been a long-serving nurse at the hospital. She was not particularly distinguished, had not in fact ever been a supervisor. But whenever a decision on patient care came up on her floor, Nurse Bryan would ask, "Are we doing the best we can do to help this patient?" Patients on Nurse Bryan's floor did better and recovered faster. Gradually over the years, the whole hospital had learned to adopt what came to be known as "Nurse Bryan's Rule"; had learned, in other words, to ask, "Are we really making the best contribution to the purpose of this hospital?"

Though Nurse Bryan herself had retired almost ten years earlier, the standards she had set still made demands on people who in terms of training and position were her superiors. (Drucker, 1967)

The application of Nurse Bryan's rule to decisions a supervisor has to make will no doubt substantially improve the quality of those decisions.

If the first five steps of the Lyles Method have been completed satisfactorily, your course of action should be fairly sound. All the unnecessary frills should have been trimmed away, possible problems uncovered and accounted for, and the plan should be ready for implementation. Before attempting to carry it out, however, one should implement the final step. In short, the proposed plan must be communicated to those who may be affected by it.

Step 6: Communicate

Overall effectiveness in problem solving and decision making is a function of both quality and acceptance. The course of action chosen must be a good one. However, no matter how good the solution, if it is not accepted by those who must support it and act to achieve the final result, the end product will be failure. The preceding steps concern activities oriented toward developing high-quality solutions. This step, however, covers issues related to gaining acceptance for those solutions to achieve the optimum final results.

Many excellent action plans have failed in the past because they were improperly communicated. Everything is meaningless unless it is acted on responsibly by others and the desired results are achieved. To avoid failure due to poor communication, one should follow these guidelines:

1. Do your homework—prepare so your ideas can be communicated in a hard-hitting presentation.
2. Present the proposal formally, no matter whom you are presenting to or how informal your relationship might be.
3. Include in your proposal actions that will benefit the people to whom you are making your proposal. This step will provide them with motivation and encourage them to respond favorably to the proposal.
4. Do not violate lines of authority, but make sure your plan to communicate will carry your proposal to *all* those who will participate in approving your idea.

Figure 7.5 shows a format that can be helpful in developing a plan to communicate.

1. Who will be affected by this action? How will they be affected?

   _____

   _____

   _____

   _____

   _____

2. Who do we need support from for success? What type of support?

   _____

   _____

   _____

   _____

   _____

3. What benefits can be identified that will accrue to those affected and to those whose support is needed for successful implementation? Be sure the benefits identified are benefits from *their* point of view.

   To those affected?   To those whose support is needed?

   _____   _____

   _____   _____

   _____   _____

   _____   _____

   _____   _____

4. How will you test the effectiveness of your communications?

   _____

   _____

   _____

   _____

   _____

   _____

Figure 7.5. Plan to communicate.

Now the plan is ready to be implemented. However, several issues to consider in this area are discussed in detail in the following section.

Step 7: Implement

To cause something to happen, you must change something. It is impossible to implement any course of action and not have something change as a result. Consequently, certain activities must be disrupted or discontinued and/or new ones must commence. But most important, it means that after you have initiated action, the situation will be different. This simple idea is often overlooked by supervisors. This oversight is reflected in comments such as, "Well, let's do it, but be careful not to make any waves." Or: "Let's get this done with as little disturbance as possible." This is the wrong focus of attention. A certain amount of disruptiveness will accompany any change. This is not bad, it is merely a fact of life. The key is to create exactly the right amount of disruption. The following guidelines should facilitate successful implementation of your action plan with the minimum amount of adverse disruption and the maximum amount of success.

1. Always implement changes from the top down.
2. Always start with the best first. Build on strengths rather than weaknesses.
3. Set your own example.
4. Remember, people cannot be motivated to do something they do not know how to do. If new knowledge or skills are required, provide opportunities for people to learn them.
5. Recognize and reward desired performance early.
6. Pace implementation so that timing is consistent with the needs of your plan. Do not try to do everything at once.
7. Provide coaching and follow-up assistance.
8. Be persistent.

When implementing, you should also establish methods for monitoring and controlling the performance of those who are carrying out the desired actions. The following guidelines will help to control performance related to your action plans:

1. Define progress indicators for the action plan.
2. Measure what is being done.
3. Keep track of progress toward the goal.
4. Take corrective action as necessary.
5. Give recognition for achievement.
6. Give special rewards for exceptional performance.

Perhaps the most important principle to remember in implementing action plans is to accept personal responsibility for results. Do not accept excuses and do not fall short of your goals simply because of another person's behavior. Truly effective supervisors accomplish the job despite obstacles or the interfering actions of others.

Having learned a reliable method for solving problems and making decisions, you should also understand several additional factors that can help improve your personal effectiveness.

ADDITIONAL FACTORS TO HELP IMPROVE PROBLEM-SOLVING AND DECISION-MAKING EFFECTIVENESS

Although the method presented in the preceding section is relatively simple and straightforward, the actual process of solving problems or making decisions is rarely easy. Several different variables can affect each problem or decision. In a recent study of a large number of experienced managers and supervisors, for example, the following suggestions were offered to new supervisors to help them improve problem-solving performance.

1. Anticipate problems, be alert for symptoms, and, whenever possible, head off problems with preventative action before they fully develop.
2. Adopt the habit of solving problems and making decisions. Avoid indecision, vacillation, procrastination, and rationalization, (but try to avoid handling problems or decisions when tired, preoccupied, or irritated).
3. Give problems and decisions priorities in accordance with their importance.
4. Subdivide particularly difficult problems, when appropriate, into related segments. (Often by solving one segment, the other segments more readily lend themselves to solution.)
5. Obtain all the facts you can. Discard irrelevant material, eliminate biases, challenge assumptions, and correlate all relevant material.
6. Draw affected people into the decision-making process. People who share in a decision, even if it is unpopular, are more likely to be committed to its success than if they had no part in it.
7. Assess risks and all possible consequences.
8. Allow time for incubation where possible. Set time limits and decide as promptly as possible, but avoid premature decisions.
9. Remember that often more than one choice will work equally well. Rarely is there only one ''right answer.''
10. Plan implementing actions carefully—consider the need for contingency plans and develop them when needed.
11. Accept personal responsibility for each decision you make and its consequences.

BENEFITS OF ENCOUNTERING PROBLEMS

Supervisors often have negative attitudes regarding problems. When unexpected obstacles or deviations arise, the situation can no doubt be frustrating. No one particularly enjoys being thrown off course unexpectedly when trying to accomplish meaningful and important goals. However, the positive, productive side to problems is worth noting.

Problems quite often reveal new ways of doing things and reasons for abandoning older, less efficient methods. Occasionally, they will reveal new opportunities that would have otherwise been missed. They force members of the organization to stay on their toes and to think about what is happening around them. Quite often, after a problem has been resolved, the situation improves. In essence, when problems arise, they should be approached in a rational, objective manner to see if perhaps they have not also created an opportunity to make improvements.

SUMMARY

There is no such thing as problem-free organization. Thus, problem solving will always be an essential skill for health care supervisors. Such problems occur in three categories: people, operational, and technical. The categories that are most important to health care supervisors will be people and operational.

The most important factor to remember when solving problems or making decisions is to focus on producing the desired results for the future. A good way to consistently produce positive results is to follow a logical method such as the Lyles Method described in this chapter. The seven steps in this method provide a logical framework that maintains a consistent focus on results.

REFERENCES

Drucker, P. F. *The Effective Executive*. New York: Harper & Row, 1967.

Lyles, R. I. *Practical Management Problem Solving and Decision Making*. New York: Van Nostrand Reinhold, 1982.

Chapter Eight

Managing Groups

Recall your most recent day at work. Try to review the various activities you pursued that day. While doing that, examine the following daily schedule of an Atlanta-based hospital unit manager:

7:30 A.M.	Meet for breakfast with other civic club members.
8:15 A.M.	Arrive at work; greet secretary and review mail.
8:25 A.M.	Receive phone call from superior.
8:30 A.M.	Hold monthly meeting with the employees in the unit.
9:20 A.M.	Review budget materials for upcoming meeting.
9:30–11:00 A.M.	Attend budget planning meeting with other unit directors.
11:00 A.M.	Meet with salesperson.
11:30 A.M.	Dictate several pieces of correspondence to secretary.
12–1:00 P.M.	Attend farewell luncheon for a retiring employee.
1:00 P.M.	Meet with new employee to give orientation and tour of unit.
1:45 P.M.	Go to personnel office to clarify earlier submitted paperwork.
2:15 P.M.	Meet with assistant supervisor of the unit to discuss safety issues.
3:00 P.M.	Attend film in hospital auditorium that reviews affirmative action programs.
4:30 P.M.	Jog with two other employees.
6:00 P.M.	Dinner with family.
7:30 P.M.	Attend son's baseball game; go out with neighbors.

What common thread can be seen in this description? Nearly all of this manager's time was spent in groups. In some cases, the group was small (meeting with secretary) and in others the group was larger (luncheon).

A supervisor, by definition, is involved in groups. Groups of many types are inevitable aspects in organizational life. The primary objective of a supervisor is to

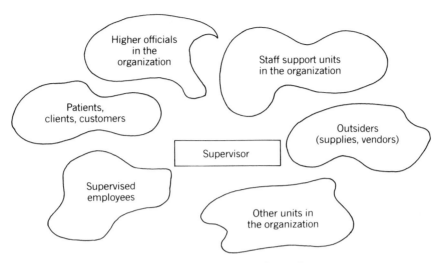

Figure 8.1. Various group relationships.

achieve organizational goals, not by working alone, but by directing the work of others—namely, the group. In addition, a supervisor relates to many other groups, some of which are depicted in Figure 8.1.

The increased interest in group behavior today is due to two factors (Anderson, 1984). The first factor is the increased technological world in which we work. This phenomenon is perhaps no more evident than in today's hospitals. Technology has advanced to such a point that no one person alone can provide the needed expertise and, therefore, groups of people must interact to provide for the patient's needs. The second concerns the acceptance of decisions. As discussed in Chapter 4, today's management literature advocates leadership styles that involve people in decision making. If more people are involved in the decision-making process, the decisions should be accepted more easily. Involving more people in decision making, however, obviously implies that more group processes and experiences will be seen.

In essence, the group can "make or break" the supervisor. Since the group is being depended on for performance, the supervisor must work to understand group issues and direct the energies of the group toward organizational goals, while at the same time fulfilling the needs and desires of the various members of the group.

DEFINITION OF TERMS

There are numerous definitions of what constitutes a group. This variety of definitions occurs because sociologists, psychologists, managers, and others are interested in groups. One definition that focuses on the multiple aspects of groups is the following: "A collection of two or more people who are interdependent and interact with one another for the purpose of performing to attain a common goal or objective'' (Ivancevich et al., 1977, p. 182). This definition highlights the critical aspects that distinguish a genuine group from just an assembly of people such as one might find at a football game. One characteristic concerns the goal-directed behavior. In other words, the group is pursuing a common goal. Second, the group interacts. Lastly, the performance dimension is emphasized.

Other terms used in this chapter are as follows:

- *Formal group*—a group that is organizationally sanctioned by the structuring of the various units.
- *Temporary group*—a meeting or committee.
- *Informal group*—any group that is not a formal or temporary group.
- *Orientation*—a period when the group is starting its work.
- *Internal problem solving*—a period of activity that is conducted during which the group begins the activities actually assigned to it.
- *Goal-based performance*—the period during which the group is actually performing on the assigned tasks of the group.
- *Cohesiveness*—the degree to which the group is united.

BENEFITS OF MANAGING GROUPS

The benefits associated with proper management of groups can be examined from two viewpoints—those benefits accruing to the individual and those accruing to the organization (Bedian & Glueck, 1983).

We have seen in earlier chapters that all people have needs. Many of these needs can be satisfied when a person joins a group. One need that people have is to socialize or *affiliate*. Groups can provide the vehicle through which people interact and share personal and work-related problems. People also like to be accepted and work groups provide the basis for this acceptance.

People also join groups to satisfy recognition and ego needs. Nurses, hospital administrators, and doctors all feel loyalty to their groups and identify with other members of their group. Bedian and Glueck (1983) describe this benefit in the following way:

> Whether people identify themselves as teachers, hospital administrators, or engineers, work groups are a primary source of recognition and esteem for most people. Through work groups, individuals attain identification, recognition, and maintain self-esteem. Others may not understand what a biochemist does, but a biochemists' co-workers know and provide necessary feedback. (p. 553)

Groups also provide benefits to people by helping to satisfy their power and security needs. Through its support, the group provides members with a sense of power against ''attacks'' by outsiders.

From the organizational standpoint, at least three benefits can be seen. The group helps to orient new employees to the organization, unit, and specific work setting. Norms, expectations, values, and attitudes are conveyed to the newcomer because the group wants to remain united. The newcomers tends to conform because of the various needs for security and affiliation, as described above.

A second benefit to the organization, which we briefly described earlier, is that the group actually accomplishes the job. No one person in any organization could perform all the complex and varied tasks. The group not only directly performs the work but can also assist the supervisor in such areas as training.

The third benefit to the organization derives from improved decision making. Group decisions are in general better than individual ones. A few of the advantages of group-based decisions are as follows (Bedian & Glueck, 1983):

- Acceptance of decisions is at a higher level than would be the case if an individual made the decision.
- Coordination required is reduced as the decision is implemented.
- Necessary communication is reduced when the decision is implemented.
- More alternatives are considered when a group is involved.
- More information is processed.

There can be some disadvantages of using groups in decision making (Anderson, 1984). At times, pressure exists to conform to the wishes of the group. Sometimes a group compromises too early and merely accepts a satisfactory solution rather than searching for the best alternative. If hierarchical or status differentials exist in a group, those lower in the hierarchy or implied status may feel intimidated by the presence of those higher. Hostile groups also may resort to "winning" rather than trying to reach the best solution. In general, the benefits to individuals and organizations outweigh the disadvantages; thus the evidence suggests that managers and supervisors should learn more about group management.

HOW SUPERVISORS RELATE TO GROUPS

Supervisors relate to groups in several different ways, as indicated in Figure 8.2. We will briefly describe these types of groups in this section, and then discuss in detail how to work successfully with these groups in a later section.

A *formal group* is one that is sanctioned by the organization and stems from the efforts to place people in various units or departments. Certain jobs and activities have to be accomplished. These units and departments tend to be reasonably permanent and use legitimate power in terms of rules, procedures, and policies to accomplish end desires.

Informal groups arise naturally and are based more on friendships, interests, mutual needs, or physical proximity. As we will see in a later section, the informal group can either contribute to or interfere with organizational and personal goal achievement.

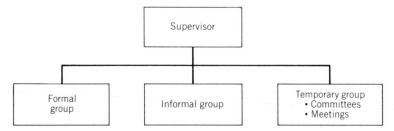

Figure 8.2. Ways of supervisory interaction with groups.

Two other ways through which supervisors interact with groups are through temporary groups (committees and meetings). We will discuss effective practices regarding each in a later section.

WHY PEOPLE JOIN GROUPS

Using the threefold classification for groups in the preceding sections, we can see that the reasons for joining groups differ. People join the formal group—the department or unit—to secure a position. In other words, you must join the formal organizational unit to earn the salary and other benefits that accompany employment. The reasons people join informal groups are quite intriguing and have been summarized by Shaw (1981). Interpersonal attraction, group activities, group goals, group membership, and instrumental benefits are some of these reasons. People join the temporary groups—committee members and meeting attendees—because they have been asked, told, or volunteered.

For instance, something about another person or other group members "attracts" a person to the group. Merely being close to a group for a period of time increases the probability that some basis of attraction will result. People with similar tastes, attitudes, and values are "attracted" to one another. Physical features and intellectual features draw people together. Essentially, the issue here is that a person sees something in the other group members at the personal level that causes this person to want to join the group.

Another reason for joining a group is that the group's activities are of interest to the person who is considering joining. People join groups to hike, play bridge, jog, discuss books, poetry, and music, and experience other forms of recreational or vocational benefit. The interpersonal factor may be nonexistent, but the interest in the activity is strong enough to cause a person to join.

A related reason is that the goals of the group appeal to the joining person. A relevant example today is the MADD group—Mothers Against Drunk Driving. People join not because of interpersonal factors, but because they agree with the goals of the group.

Another reason, which we addressed earlier, is that the mere act of being a member of a group can fulfill individual needs for security, status, and affiliation.

Finally, the indirect benefits that one may accrue by being a member of a certain group are incentives for joining a group. For example, some people join civic clubs and social clubs primarily for the contacts that they may make and such contacts might be "instrumental" in furthering their careers. Obviously, we are not saying this is the only reason people join civic and social clubs.

The supervisor should be aware that people join groups for various reasons and that groups can fulfill various needs and wants of individuals in groups. You may want to perform an exercise with yourself. First, list all the groups of which you are a member. Be sure to include work and nonwork settings. Then see if you can determine or recall the primary reason why you joined each group. Do you notice any pattern in the various reasons? In a similar fashion, think of all the groups you have left. Again, be sure to include work and nonwork groups and complete the rest of the exercise.

STAGES OF GROUP DEVELOPMENT

A group evolves through a number of stages as it moves from being a collection of people to a united, high-performing, cohesive group. Various approaches to group development, described by different authors, are summarized in Table 8.1). After reviewing these different approaches, as well as others, we noticed three major stages through which groups may move:

- Orientation
- Internal problem solving
- Goal-based performance

In the first step, group members are cautious because they do not know one another. Structure, rules, and guidelines are missing, and the group is searching for direction. Group members are asking questions similar to the following:

- Can I trust this group?
- What will I obtain from this group?
- What will I have to do as a member of this group?

In essence, group members are "feeling each other out" to determine expectations, acceptable behavior, and structure.

In the second stage, the groups begin to experience conflict. Various subgroups begin to form and questions of group leadership arise. Arguments are likely to be generated regarding the techniques and mechanics of the group's operations. The labeling of this stage—internal problem solving—means that the group's efforts are directed more to the group itself rather than focused on the primary goal(s) that gave rise to the group in the first place. This step may be referred to as "getting the bugs out."

Table 8.1

**Different Approaches
to the Formation of Groups**

Orientation
Internal problem solving
Growth and Productivity
Evaluation and Control (Ivancevich et al., 1977)

Forming
Storming
Norming
Performing (Griffin, 1984)

Mutual acceptance
Decision making
Motivation
Control (Donnelly et al., 1981)

Forming
Storming
Initial integration
Total integration (Schermerhorn, 1984)

Membership
Subgrouping
Confrontation
Individual differentiation
Collaboration (Cohen et al., 1984)

In the third stage, the group focuses on the problem at hand. The efforts of the group are directed toward achieving the individual and organizational goals and the infighting of the group is no longer an issue. The group members will still raise issues, question one another, and speak openly about concerns, but the thrust is complementary rather than antagonistic.

Every supervisor prefers to have the various groups at the third stage, but stages one and two should not be rushed. According to Cohen et al. (1984), the three major concerns are as follows:

> One danger is the temptation to avoid conflict by patching things over prematurely before the issues are fully explored and by establishing norms against rocking the boat or raising controversial subjects. When this happens the disagreements and any associated bad feelings among members go underground, ready to affect future business in often indirect and insidious ways.
>
> A second danger is that disagreement and conflict are dealt with strictly through power, so that one individual or one subgroup "wins" and others "lose"; the issue remains unresolved. Someone emerges as a loser, often resulting in

either withdrawal or warfare. Withdrawal reduces the group's resources and is hardly a source of satisfaction and growth for the individuals involved. Warfare, which typically is carried over to the next task facing the group, is a sure way to guarantee lowered productivity and energies devoted to attack and self-defense rather than growth. A third danger is merely a continuation of the struggle and a lack of energy for any new projects. (p. 145)

In the next section, various factors that give rise to increased performance and cohesion will be discussed.

WHAT CAUSES GROUPS TO BE MORE COHESIVE AND PERFORMING

Before we discuss the factors causing higher group cohesion, it may be beneficial to describe what happens when groups are more cohesive. According to Griffin (1984):

> In general as groups become more cohesive, their members tend to interact more frequently, conform more to group norms, and become more satisfied with the group. Cohesiveness may also influence group performance. (p. 460)

The use of the word "may" in terms of performance is because of the interaction between cohesion and performance norms. Seashore (1984), who conducted research with groups and found that some groups had high productivity levels while others had low productivity, concluded the following:

> If a group felt confident in management, it would enforce a high production level. If it had a poor opinion of management, its production was uniformly low. Interestingly, group morale was high in either case. (p. 332)

In other words, we have the following four situations:

- Low cohesion, low performance norms
- Low cohesion, high performance norms
- High cohesion, high performance norms
- High cohesion, low performance norms

In the third case, the highly cohesive groups would produce at high levels. In the fourth situation, the group is united, but performance will not be high. Such a situation can be illustrated when a work force is unionized and cohesive but, because of opposition to management, the group may intentionally decide to withhold performance.

Figure 8.3 summarizes the factors that impact cohesiveness (Ivancevich et al., 1977). As can be seen, each factor either increases or decreases cohesiveness, depending on the way the factor is used.

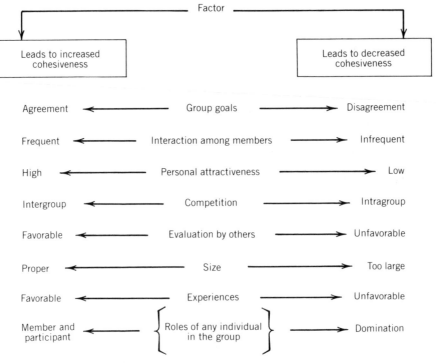

Figure 8.3. Factors impacting group cohesiveness. From *Organization Behavior and Performance* by Ivancevich, J. M., Szilagyi, A. D., and Wallace, M. J. Copyright © 1977 by Scott, Foresman and Company. Reprinted by permission.

- *Group goals:* If the group agrees on the goals, the members will rally behind the efforts of the group and be more loyal to the group. Disagreement leads to conflict and infighting.
- *Interaction among members:* If the group members have frequent chance for interaction, there is an increased likelihood that they will become more united in their loyalties, interests, and actions. A supervisor should, in turn, have meetings and arrange facilities so that group members can interact more frequently.
- *Personal attractiveness:* As discussed earlier, people join groups at times because the activities and goals of the group are of interest or have some attraction for the newcomer. People can also become more united and cohesive because of the same factors. The people become attracted to one another and "the key factor . . . is that they enjoy working with each other" (Lott & Lott, 1965).
- *Competition:* Competition with other groups—intercompetition—tends to bring the group members together. A good example of how this factor works

can be seen in sports teams and sales contests among various units in organizations. On the other hand, too much competition within the group—intracompetition—leads to conflict, infighting, jealousy, and dissension.

- *Evaluation by others:* If the group has been evaluated favorably by some other important person or group, such recognition unites the group by appealing to its collective ego and status needs. Conversely, an unfavorable evaluation can lead to trying to find the person responsible for the action or blaming other group members, which ultimately disunites the group.
- *Size:* The common sense message regarding this factor is that groups can become too large. If the group becomes too large, subgroups begin to form that may have interests different from the overall group. In addition, the chance for interaction decreases as too many group members vie for the limited time and contacts that are available.
- *Experiences:* If the group has pleasant experiences together, such experiences feed on each other and the members look forward to future contacts with the group, which increases interactions and makes the group even further united. Conversely, unpleasant experiences cause members to begin to reject the group and become more alienated.
- *Role of any individual in the group:* If one or more group members dominate the discussions, activities, and processes of the group, cohesiveness does not develop properly. Such domination interferes with the rapport and positive interactions of the group.

If a cohesive group provides member satisfaction, as well as benefits to the organization, the supervisor is then challenged to consider factors such as those covered in this section to move a group from being merely a collection of people to a highly cohesive work group.

McGregor (1960), who developed the Theory X and Theory Y approach to leadership and a major contributor to management thought, indentified eleven characteristics of more effective groups.

1. The group atmosphere should be relaxed and informal.
2. Member participation in group discussions should be high.
3. The group members should fully understand and accept the objectives of the group.
4. The group members should be open with one another and should listen to one another's ideas.
5. Conflict and disagreement is managed and ''win-win'' solutions should be sought. Conflict should not be ''swept under the rug.''
6. Decisions should be reached by some consensus method.
7. Group discussion should raise issues and concerns but should not reach the level of personal attacks on other members.
8. Group members should feel free to question the direction in which the group is moving.

9. Task assignments within the groups should be clearly delineated.

10. The leader of the group should use more of a "joining" style.

11. The group should be sensitive to monitor its own performance.

MANAGING SPECIAL TYPES OF GROUPS

As we indicated in Figure 8.2, supervisors interact with formal, informal, and temporary groups. Other chapters in this book have focused on the formal aspects of the organization. In this section, we will discuss managerial issues associated with informal and temporary groups (meetings and committees).

Informal groups

Although more elaborate definitions exist of what constitutes an informal group, the easiest way to describe it is that any group that is not formally sanctioned by the organization is an informal one. Informal groups are inevitable consequences of organizational life. It is important for supervisors to accept, recognize, and use the informal group. There is nothing inherently dysfunctional about informal groups. Informal groups can be contributing elements in organizations or they can be obstacles and negative in nature. The difference results from the way the supervisor uses the informal group.

Davis (1961) suggests that informal groups are formed for five reasons. The first basis is for friendship reasons. All of us have affiliation and belonging needs and the group allows us to fulfill these needs.

Second, informal groups allow people to communicate. The formal communication channels may take too long and the grapevine, "rumor mill," or other informal channel allows for the information to be shared by group members.

Informal groups also help to control the pace of work. The informal group can signal to a new employee what amount of work constitutes a good day's work.

Informal groups fulfill people's prestige, status, and ego needs. People can be recognized and feel important in a group, whereas they may not in the formal organization.

Lastly, it is through the informal group that the organizational culture is maintained. Rites, values, traditions, and heroes are set by the informal organization.

Many of the guidelines for managing the formal group are also appropriate for the informal group. Several additional suggestions can be made regarding the management of the informal group:

- Accept the informal group and work through it; do not try to abolish it.
- Learn as much as you can about the informal group.
- Respect the group's standards and norms unless they are contrary and interfere with those preferred.
- Be fair to the group and emphasize performance.

- Involve the group in decision making if there is an indication that the group can provide constructive input.
- Support the informal leaders of the group and use, not abuse, them.
- Try to make the group more cohesive and work toward organizational goals and objectives.

If these suggestions are not followed, the informal leaders of the group may initiate actions and adopt practices that are contrary to the formal goals and objectives.

Temporary Groups

Meetings

Supervisors and managers spend a considerable amount of their time in meetings. Meetings are similar to informal groups in that there is nothing inherently good or bad about them—it all depends on how effectively the meetings are managed. Meetings can have positive outcomes but may at times make people feel that their time has been wasted. Supervisors will sometimes call meetings of their own and at other times be required to attend someone else's meeting. Regardless of the situation, the following guidelines should prove beneficial (Huse, 1982):

- The formal leader of the meeting should be a good listener and be prepared to work with the informal leaders of the group.
- An advance agenda for the meeting should be prepared and distributed.
- The consensus approach to decision making should be used.
- The size of the committee should typically range from five to ten members.
- The physical surroundings should provide for a good meeting atmosphere.
- The meeting leader should periodically summarize the position of the group and keep the discussion directed toward the agenda items.
- The leader should realize that feelings, emotions, and processes are important in addition to the task requirements of the meeting.

Committees

Committees can also be effective or ineffective as ways of reaching a group-based decision. The preceding guidelines for meetings would also apply to committee meetings. In addition, the following guidelines are appropriate for committees:

- Choose only those members whose involvement is needed.
- Limit the size of the committee.
- Define clear goals and objectives for the committee.
- Appoint an effective formal leader.

SUMMARY

Groups are the natural result of bringing people together in organizations. Supervisors cannot accomplish their goals without the involvement of various work groups. Remember the following points on managing groups:

- The individual members and the organization can benefit from positive group experiences.
- People join groups to satisfy various needs.
- Groups help the organization by orienting newcomers, ensuring that work is accomplished, and rendering improved decision making.
- Supervisors relate to formal, informal, and temporary groups (meetings and committees).
- People join groups because of interpersonal attraction, the activities of the group, the group's goals, and the membership benefits.
- Groups move through stages of orientation, internal problem solving, and goal-based performance.
- A cohesive group is preferred if its performance norms are high and positive.
- Informal groups form because of friendship, communications, work pace, need fulfillment, and organizational culture reasons.
- Meetings and committees can be good or bad for the organization, and guidelines should be followed.

REFERENCES

Anderson, C. R. *Management Skills, Functions, and Organization Performance.* Dubuque, IW: Brown, 1984.

Bedian, A. G., & Glueck, W. F. *Management.* New York: Dryden Press, 1983.

Cohen, A.R., Fink, S. L., Gadon, H., & Willits, R. D. *Effective Behavior in Organizations.* Homewood, IL: Irwin, 1984.

Davis, K. *Human Relations at Work.* New York: McGraw-Hill, 1962.

Donnelly, J. H., Jr., Gibson, J. L., & Ivancevich, J. M. *Fundamentals of Management: Functions, Behavior, Models.* Plano, TX: Business Publications, 1981.

Griffin, R. W. *Management.* Boston: Houghton Mifflin, 1984.

Huse, E. F. *Management.* New York: West, 1982.

Ivancevich, J. M., Szilagyi, A. D., Jr., & Wallace, M. J. *Organizational Behavior and Human Performance.* Santa Monica, CA: Goodyear, 1977.

Lott, A. J., & Lott, B. E. (1965). "Group cohesiveness as interpersonal attraction: a review of relationships with antecedent and consequent variables." *Psychological Bulletin,* 259–309.

McGregor, D. *The Human Side of Enterprise.* New York: McGraw-Hill, 1960.

Schermerhorn, J. R. *Management for Productivity.* New York: Wiley, 1984.

Seashore, S. F. ''Group Cohesiveness in the Industrial Work Group.'' In Louis E. Boone & David L. Kurtz (Eds.), *Principles of Management*. New York: Random House, 1984.

Shaw, M. E. *Group Dynamics: The Psychology of Small Group Behavior*. New York: McGraw-Hill, 1981.

Chapter Nine

Time Management

When was the last time you said, "I didn't have enough time?" Was it yesterday, last week, last month, or perhaps as recently as this morning?

"I did not have enough time." Think of what this means. Consider the significance of this statement and how misleading it is. The statement is completely fraudulent, misleading, and deceptive.

How much time did you have yesterday? There is no way you could have had any more or any less time than anyone else. We each have 24 hours to spend each day. There are 168 hours every week, and 52 weeks each year. No more, no less.

There is nothing any one of can do to obtain more or fewer hours in a day, more or fewer hours in a week, or more or fewer weeks in a year. So to say that there was not enough time yesterday or last week or last month or at any time is to mislead.

The nature of time and the way we talk about time raise two important issues that must be understood if we are to make effective use of our time: (1) time as a resource; and (2) personal responsibility for time use.

TIME AS A RESOURCE

The previous chapters discussed the various resources for which supervisors are responsible. These primarily include money, equipment, facilities, and people. Another resource equally important is the resource of time. Without time, we can accomplish nothing.

But time differs from other resources. Money comes and goes at different rates. The way we account for it makes a significant difference regarding its usefulness to the organization. Equipment and facilities vary from location to location, and their quality is affected by time and use. People—as human resources—possess as many different characteristics and traits as there are individuals. Each is unique. Consequently, we must be flexible in style to gain their maximum contribution. Time, however, possesses none of these characteristics. Time itself is always the same. Each second is identical to the last and every minute is an exact copy of its predecessor. Time is distributed at a finite and predictable rate. The availability of time is the same today as it was last week and will be next week. We cannot do anything about availability of time nor can we alter its quality.

Thus talking about time management is talking in deceptive and misleading terms. How can we manage something we cannot affect? We can manage human resources because we can influence people by changing their behavior, developing their skills, and causing them to use more or less of their potential. We can also manipulate financial resources and modify equipment and facilities, but we simply cannot affect time.

At best, we can *manage ourselves in relation to time*. Thus, rather than time management, we should use the phrase "self-management in relation to time." This raises the issue of personal responsibility for time use.

PERSONAL RESPONSIBILITY FOR TIME USE

Language often drives behavior. When we use certain phrases to describe different situations, our behavior is pushed in those directions without our complete awareness of what is happening. This phenomenon is widespread when the topic is time. Consider the underlying assumptions that are reinforced when a person states: "I didn't have enough time." The first implication is that time is to blame. "What could I do? There simply wasn't enough time to go around." In other words, we're saying, "Don't blame me, blame time." Time is to blame. Since time is to blame, I don't have to accept the responsibility for not achieving the things I should have. Carried to the extreme, this can create a frustrating situation in which no one is willing to accept responsibility for his or her own performance.

In fact, in one clinic the situation became so intolerable that the supervisor called the entire staff together and established a rather unique rule. She said that from that day forward no one could say "I didn't have enough time." Instead of using this worn-out phrase, henceforth the correct reply would be, "I chose not to spend my time that way." Then there would be no confusion about the focus of responsibility. Although this approach may sound more drastic than it actually is, the point was made. The chaos in the clinic began to diminish as people accepted personal responsibility for using time.

Since we can do nothing about time and time can do nothing about itself, who is responsible? Each of us must make the appropriate use of time by choosing to spend our time in ways that are most useful. We must use available time to achieve our most important goals.

Thus the essence of effective management of self in relation to time is to make good decisions about how our time is spent. At any particular instant, there may be unlimited choices. We might face the prospect of choosing between work and play or between social or family activity. It might be time to eat, sleep, bathe, rest, take a walk, mow the lawn, wash the dishes, jog, write a letter, or read a book. At various times, managers, subordinates, family, friends, neighbors, colleagues, or even strangers might make demands on our time. The level of these demands fluctuates over time. Although we can rarely control the level or the frequency of the demands, we can control how we respond to them. We control the decisions we make about how we spend our time, and we decide how we will manage ourselves in relation to time. The essence of time management is not managing time, it is managing self.

Self-Management Techniques

What is time? According to Lakein (1972), ''Time is life and life is time. If you waste your time, you are wasting your life.'' The implication is that if people want to make optimum use of the time that is available to them, it is important for each to know what he or she wants out of life. In other words, establishing goals in life is the place to start.

How can anyone know what is important today, if they do not know what is important overall? How can a person possibly know whether doing one thing is more important than another if they do not know what is important to them to begin with? The key to effective time use is being able to make the right decision about how time should be spent when numerous choices exist.

In the absence of personal goals, all time management techniques become manipulation. Rather than *managing* in relation to time, a person is simply manipulating activities in relation to time. When this happens, there is no true reward. Results will be sporadic and many times meaningless. Frustration and dissatisfaction will once again reappear with the realization that little of true importance is being accomplished.

Activities by themselves are not important or unimportant. Importance is determined by a person's goals. There is no such thing as an efficient or effective activity by itself. Activity acquires meaning through the goals that lie behind it. Thus all time management activity, to bring meaning to the person who is using it, must start with goals.

A simple yet effective self-management process is outlined in Figure 9.1. Notice that the starting point is setting goals. After goals are established, we establish priorities. Using goals and priorities as a background, we assess our time use. Tools and techniques are then used to leverage our time into more effective and efficient use. Finally, we periodically reassess or reevaluate the process which may then lead to new goal setting. Let us now examine each of these steps in more detail.

The first step is to set goals. What do you want from life? Within that context, what do you want to achieve during your career? Even more specific, what do you want to achieve in your current job with the most immediate challenges you face? Think of the short- (six months to a year) and long-range (more than a year) goals, including post-retirement activities. Goals describe what is important to you in life, career, and job.

After setting goals, establish priorities. While goals tell what is *important,* priorities focus on *urgency.* Priorities tell us how soon things must be done or at least in what order activities should be undertaken. Although all goals may be important, they may vary widely in urgency. Some should be accomplished as soon as possible, while others may be delayed, In fact, some may even benefit if they are delayed.

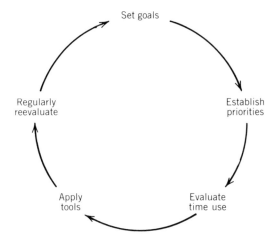

Figure 9.1. Self-management process.

Once goals and priorities are set, it is time to assess current time use. The best way to do this is to keep a time diary for several days. Table 9.1 gives an example of a typical time diary format. Half-hour time intervals are best for most supervisors in health care organizations because of the nature of their work. Since activities vary from day-to-day, data for one day's work are not enough to obtain a true picture of how time is being used. Data should be collected for at least two days, preferably three or four. It is also important to complete the diary during the time in which time use is being assessed. Record events as they happen. Do not try to list them the next day or the next week since too many details will be forgotten and the assessment will be meaningless.

After assessing time use, one then applies the right techniques to leverage activities into more productive areas. The goal of all time management techniques is to help the individual make better personal decisions regarding time use. The key is to decide to do the things that are most important when discretionary time is available. None of us has complete control over all of our time. The key for effective time use is to make the right decisions when, in fact, we have control over the time that we are using.

The next step is to reassess periodically or reevaluate goals, priorities, and time use. Time management is a dynamic, ongoing process that sustains itself over time. Goals, priorities, and decisions regarding how to use our time will change. It is thus important for us to critique our time use and to make sure that we are doing the things that are most important to us at any particular time.

To summarize thus far then, it is important to remember several points. First, it is self-management, not time management, that is the key to effective use of time. Second, to be effective at self-management in relation to time, we must follow a logical management process. Third, a logical management process starts with establishing goals and setting priorities. It continues with assessing time use and using

Table 9.1

| Date: _____ Day of Week: _____ ||||
Time	Activity	Time	Activity
7:30		1:00	
8:00		1:30	
8:30		2:00	
9:00		2:30	
9:30		3:00	
10:00		3:30	
10:30		4:00	
11:00		4:30	
11:30		5:00	
12:00		5:30	

the time techniques that we are aware of to make better decisions regarding the use of our time. And finally, time management is an ongoing, dynamic process that sustains itself over time and must receive constant attention.

To sustain this ongoing attention, a supervisor must be personally organized. In other words, organization of self is a prerequisite to carrying out effective time management techniques.

Self-Organization

Time waits for no one, including the supervisor. The supervisor, therefore, should spend time like money. Time should be allocated to those activities that yield the greatest return. The best way to ensure consistently good returns is to be personally organized. The following guidelines will help in becoming organized on a personal level:

1. At the end of each day, decide what priorities must be carried forward and write them down.
2. Arrive at work early (at least 20 minutes) and plan your day.
3. Develop a job plan for your job and for the people who work for you.
4. Prepare for your absence and that of others in order that productivity can be maintained during vacations, illness, or injuries.
5. Delegate routine work to responsible workers.
6. Schedule as much as possible. This includes meetings, personal conferences, and telephone calls.
7. Complete the most important work of the day first.
8. Allow time each day for emergencies, interruptions, and other unexpected but legitimate requests for your time.

The only one of these items that may require further elaboration is the development of a job plan. The following section describes this activity.

Development of Job Plan

First, specify the key job responsibilities. What must be done to satisfy the requirements of the job? Be sure to identify the nonroutine, as well as the routine, activities that must be fulfilled.

Next, list the times at which the activities must occur. When must these actions be taken? Consider special responsibilities together with any actions that should be taken daily, weekly, monthly, quarterly, semi-annually, or annually.

Finally, include an explanation of how these responsibilities are to be accomplished. How should each duty be carried out? These guidelines should address each item in detail so that others will understand well enough to be able to perform the job without much supervision. Exhibits and samples should be included as needed. Refer to Figure 9.2 to see a format for developing a job plan. Notice that the responsibilities appear in the first column, the timing for fulfilling those responsibilities is entered in the second column, and the instructions for carrying them out appear in the third.

Several additional items that could also be assembled in the job plan might include the following:

- A list of internal and external contacts. The list should include name, title, location, telephone number, and possible reason for contacting this person.

Key job responsibilities	Time at which it must occur	How responsibility should be carried out

Figure 9.2. Format for developing job plan.

- A list of terms or words peculiar to your operation or to your department.
- Explanation of files, which includes a diagram and sufficient information so that different files can be located with relative ease.
- An organization chart, which lists the lines of responsibility and authority for the immediate department, as well as for the organization as a whole.
- Reference sources, including a list commonly used reference materials that a person filling the job might need to locate information.

In addition to this information, people might also keep information, such as personal lists, lists of subscriptions, birthdays or special dates and events that are recognized in the group, membership rosters, travel information, and perhaps a biography of the manager. It is important that people have information readily available to them so they do not have to search and ask routine questions that they can more easily answer if the information is presented to them in a simple format.

Beyond organization on a personal level, several specific activities a supervisor can use to improve the effective use of time include the following:

1. Keep extra work available to enhance productivity during periods of slack time. Avoid idle time by keeping a backlog of available work.
2. Reduce paperwork. Write replies on the letter or memo itself. Develop model letters for repetitive situations.
3. Conduct effective meetings. Set time limits, use agendas, and adhere to the time schedule.

4. Group a number of small or insignificant tasks together and complete them all at once.

5. Gather all the facts on problems before making a decision.

6. After obtaining sufficient information, be decisive.

7. Do not become emotionally involved in matters of other departments or parts of the organization that do not affect you.

8. Give clear and simple directions to workers to avoid misunderstandings.

9. Delegate as much as possible. Delegation helps other workers improve their performance and it provides more meaningful work opportunities as well as saving you time.

10. Do not procrastinate, do it now.

11. Say no when asked for work not consistent with achieving your work group's goals.

12. Look for ways to get your job and the job of your subordinates done in less time.

13. Be on time for appointments and encourage others to do the same.

14. Minimize the effect of telephone interruptions by asking interrupters to call back later. If possible, return all calls at a scheduled part of the day. Do not let phone interruptions interfere with a more important person-to-person conversation in your office.

15. Read important material only. Do not become bogged down with junk mail and do not waste time reading things that are insignificant.

16. Periodically monitor how you are spending your time by completing a simple log for several days at a time.

17. Return all phone calls.

18. Avoid unnecessary conversations. Excuse yourself to leave, stand up and move to the door when the conversation drifts from important topics, or ask to set appointments in other people's offices so you can leave when the conversation becomes irrelevant.

19. Occasionally schedule working lunches. Although not effective when many specific tasks are to be accomplished, working lunches can be beneficial when informal discussion and greater understanding of issues are the objectives.

Many health care supervisors fall into the traps of doing what they are told to do, what they like to do, or things in which they excel. This can be satisfying but, at times, it can be unproductive as well. Supervisory responsibilities extend into areas in which the supervisor does not feel confident or comfortable. Part of personal organization includes maintaining an objective focus and doing the things that need to be done, regardless of whether a supervisor either has been told or likes to do them.

Effective supervisors are initiators who know what needs to be done and then do it. An effective supervisor manages the job primarily because he or she is able to understand how to spend his or her time and is able to manage it effectively while at work. However, it is not just knowing what to do from a positive sense that makes the difference. Often in organizations, time wasters arise that interfere with the supervisor's ability to apply this time management knowledge. Let us examine some of these time wasters and how they might be handled.

Time Wasters

Wilson (1982), who conducted a survey of time management research, examined time wasters among administrators and managers at all levels in diverse organizations. As a result, he compiled a detailed list of universal time wasters. With rare exception, the following five time wasters appear at the top of every list:

1. Telephone interruptions
2. Drop-in visiting
3. Meetings (both scheduled and unscheduled)
4. Crisis
5. Lack of objectives, priorities, and deadlines

Ranking close behind these is another group of five time wasters.

1. Cluttered desk and personal disorganization
2. Ineffective delegation and involvement in routine and detail
3. Attempting too much at once and unrealistic time estimates
4. Confused responsibility and authority
5. Inadequate, inaccurate, or delayed information

The final cluster of time wasters seems to depend more on worker habits and norms, leadership styles, and organizational characteristics:

1. Indecision and procrastination
2. Lack of, or unclear, communication or instruction
3. Inability to say "no"
4. Lack of controls, standards, and progress reports
5. Fatigue and/or lack of self-discipline

These factors, according to administrators and supervisors, are preventing them from being as effective as they would like to be. Moreover, the findings are consistent with another study that Mackenzie (1972) conducted among management experts. This second study identified 35 time wasters associated with the different functions of management. These factors are illustrated in Figure 9.3.

Besides knowing that these factors affect others in positions similar to yours, you should also recognize how these factors affect you personally. Which of them have the strongest impact on you? Which of them interferes most with your effective use

35 Time Wasters by Supervisory Function

Decision Making
  Decision by committee
  Wanting all the facts
  Indecision/Procrastinating
  Snap decisions

Communicating
  Socializing
  Failure to listen
  Under/Unclear/Over-communicating
  Meetings

Controlling
  Inability to say "No"
  Overlooking poor performance
  Mistakes/Ineffective performance
  Over-control
  No standards/Progress reports
  Incomplete information
  Telephone/Visitors

Directing
  Not coping with change
  Not managing conflict
  No coordination/Teamwork
  Lack of motivation
  Ineffective delegation
  Involved in routine details
  Doing it myself

Staffing
  Personnel with problems
  Under/Over-staffed
  Untrained/Inadequate staff

Organizing
  Multiple bosses
  Confused responsibility and authority
  Duplication of effort
  Personal disorganization/Stacked desk

Planning
  Attempting too much/Unrealistic time estimates
  No self-imposed deadlines (day-dreaming)
  Fire fighting/Crisis management
  Leaving tasks unfinished
  Shifting priorities
  No objectives, priorities, or daily plan

Adapted from Mackenzie, R. A. *The Time Trap: Managing Your Way Out.* New York: American Management Association, 1972. © R. Alec Mackenzie, 1972.

Figure 9.3. Time wasters by supervisory function.

of time? To help answer these questions, Wilson (1982) developed a method for self-analysis of supervisorial effectiveness. Use it as a guide to determine which time wasters bother you the most. The following outline will guide you in your analysis.

Evaluation of Time Use Effectiveness

1. What percentage of your objectives is accomplished on time and in order of priority?

2. What percentage of self-imposed deadlines do you meet?

3. How do the results you achieve compare to the amount of effort you expend achieving them? In other words, do you spend the most amount of your time achieving the most important results?

4. How well do you control interruptions? How many interruptions do you experience per hour or per day?

5. Do you spend a certain percentage of your time each day trying to accomplish your most important objectives?

6. How often do you leave tasks unfinished?

7. Are you often frustrated by the amount of work you are trying to accomplish? How often do you feel this frustration?

8. Do you consistently have a backlog of work to be accomplished? Some backlog is good because it helps maintain productivity, but is yours appropriate for your position?

9. How many surprises do you encounter each day? How often are you surprised by events or occurrences that could or should have been anticipated?

10. What is your availability for taking on new responsibilities or responding to new challenges? How often are you sufficiently "caught up" to accept new responsibilities without hardship or undue stress?

Review your answers to these questions to determine your personal areas of strength and weakness. Areas of strength should be highlighted to be used as a springboard to future development. Areas of weakness should be investigated to determine which time wasters from the previous list or from Figure 9.2 are causing a problem. The most serious time wasters should be identified and attacked so that you may proceed with positive developments and more effective use of your time. The following section describes a number of techniques for attacking the most serious time wasters.

ELIMINATING TIME WASTERS

Again, the best place to find information on time wasters and how to handle them is in Wilson's research (1982). He has identified the time wasters by category and, through his work with administrators and supervisors, has developed numerous techniques and tools to help eliminate them from the environment. The following ideas are adapted from his time management tools and techniques check list.

Lack of Planning

Anticipatory thinking—planning ahead and making preparations to handle the future—is an effective ally for a supervisor striving to use time effectively. Planning and identifying results in advance are the keys to being personally organized and effective. The following techniques will help overcome lack of planning.

Periodically Set Goals.   Setting goals includes identifying and writing down short- and long-range life and work-related goals. It also means at least having a minimum outline of an action plan to accomplish both life goals and work goals.

Use a Time Budget.   This includes classifying your work activities into different types of work—regular, routine, created, and special—and allocating a certain percentage of your time for each. Organize your day and your week around your time budget and evaluate your actual time use compared to your time budget at the end of each week.

Write Performance Standards for Major Work Activities.   This requires identifying benchmarks of performance as a guideline concerning how long different activities should take and what the expected completion time should be.

Clearly Define Priorities.   Develop a system for prioritizing tasks, activities, and decisions so that the most important activities can be accomplished first.

Perform Tasks in the Order of Priority.   Complete the most important work first. Avoid allowing the urgent tasks to supersede the important one. Maintain a focus on what is important.

Use a daily "to do" list. The list should be in writing. Rather than list all the routine activities you hope to accomplish each day, it should list the most important things you are trying to accomplish, whether or not they will all be accomplished immediately. The list should be prioritized with estimated completion times for each activity. Remember a "to do" list is only an aid to help you decide how to use your time when discretionary time is available.

Complete Tasks on Your "To Do" List According to their Priority.   When you have discretionary time available, refer to the "to do" list to identify the most important items. Choose to do the most important item on the list.

Obtain Necessary Information before Starting a Major Project.   Avoid interrupting your own work by tracking down bits of information every few minutes, because this will only cause inconsistent work and erratic performance.

Program Variety into Your Work Routine.   Avoid allowing your work routine to become monotonous. Schedule different kinds of activities so that your thought processes stay stimulated and your work remains interesting.

Schedule Time for Unscheduled Activities.   On the basis of past experience, determine what level of unscheduled activities you are required to handle on a regular basis. Allow some flextime in your schedule so that you can respond to unscheduled work demands with minimal disruption.

Drop-in Visitors

Drop-in visitors can include anyone. People from inside or outside the organization who drop in unexpectedly can create frustrating and dysfunctional interruptions in the normal work flow. It is important to note that even though patients or people who use our services may drop in unexpectedly, they should always be treated pleasantly and positively so that neither they nor we forget why we are in business. Here are some ways to handle unscheduled visitors.

Discourage Unscheduled Visits.   Set up work routines and work habits that make it difficult for someone to interrupt. Let people know that the best time for visiting might be prior to commencement of the shift, during a break, during lunch hour, or following the completion of the daily work schedule.

Establish an Ending Time at the Beginning of Such Visits.   This technique can be done informally as well as formally. Perhaps a casual remark such as: "It's good to see you, I have about 5 minutes that we can visit," would be useful.

Bring Closure to Conversations after Business Has Been Addressed.   Develop the habit of saying, "It's been nice visiting with you, but I have pressing projects I must return to," or "I'd like to visit more with you in the future, maybe we'll have some time soon," or these methods can be nonverbal like simply standing, asking to be excused, or moving toward the door in cases where the conversation seems to be dragging.

Designate Someone to Screen Visitors.   This person may be a secretary, receptionist, or someone whose desk or work station is in a convenient location to screen out visitors who lack urgent agendas for discussion. Reorganizing the work setting or the work environment to keep people out is beneficial.

Meet with Visitors in the Reception Area.   When visitors, especially drop-in visitors, are invited into the office, this situation often results in sharing a cup of coffee and settling in for an extended visit. Frequently, such visits can be kept to a minimum if they are conducted standing up in the reception areas, since the person who is being interrupted can always leave to attend another appointment or a meeting or to respond to some other priority that may have arisen.

Visit Standing Up.   The simple act of sitting down and ''getting comfortable'' will double or triple the time that would otherwise be required for a drop-in visit. By not allowing this to happen, the duration of the visit can be kept to a minimum.

Telephone

Telephones can be one of the greatest time savers in the modern work environment. It is unfortunate that such a tremendous tool of convenience can at the same time be such a tremendous time waster. Time wasted from telephones results from disorganized phone calls, telephone interruptions, or failure to realize the true potential of the telephone as a tool. The following are some techniques for improving telephone use.

After Greetings, Make Business the First Item of Discussion.   As pleasant as it may seem, talking about the weather, outside interests, or social activities waste time on the job. On-the-job phone conversations should be focused toward work activities.

Bring Closure to Conversations after Business Has Been Conducted.   Because the telephone plays such a tremendous part in our social lives, we have a tendency to allow this social dimension to carry over into the work setting. Conscious effort is required to weed this out of our behavioral patterns and maintain focus and efficient use of our telephone time.

Limit 90 Percent of Your Calls to Three Minutes of Duration.   It is important to check your telephone calls periodically to see if they are extending beyond reasonable limits. Most on-the-job conversations that are required can easily be conducted in three minutes or less. If most of your calls are not staying within this three-minute limitation, chances are you are wasting a significant percentage of your telephone time.

Use Conference Calls in Place of Meetings.   With all the new features of the modern telephone services, it is easy to set up conference calls and to use joint calls rather than spend the time traveling to and from different meeting places.

Use The Telephone Instead of Letters or Memorandums.   It is much easier to pick up the telephone to send your message than it is to write a memo, have it typed, proofread it, package it, and send it. If it is necessary to keep track of the information that is transmitted by a telephone, keep a note pad next to the telephone and jot down key ideas and the dates and times for certain telephone conversations.

Cluster and Return Telephone Calls at a Set Time Each Day.   Rather than make phone calls at random intervals during the day, make all your return calls at once. Set aside your telephone time for the occasions when people are most likely to be in their offices or reachable and when you have the least probability of experiencing interference.

Gather the Information You Need Prior to Returning Calls.   Anticipate information needs prior to telephone conversations. Organize the information so that it can be transmitted crisply and in a businesslike manner.

Meetings

Like the telephone, meetings can be either tremendous time savers or tremendous time wasters, depending on how they are used. One only needs to multiply the number of people attending the meeting by the amount of time wasted to gain an appreciation for the true expenditure of effort that is wasted in meetings. For example, if six people are attending the meeting and ten minutes of that meeting are wasted, we have wasted not only ten minutes, but also one work hour of productivity. If six people waste an hour, they have wasted almost a full workday's worth of productivity. Thus meetings should be both efficient and effective. The following guidelines suggest ways to achieve that goal.

Question the Necessity of Every Meeting.   Do not schedule meetings that are not needed and do not conduct regularly scheduled staff meetings, unless there is a valid reason for doing so. If there is no important business to transact, cancel the meeting.

Question Your Own Involvement in Meetings You Do Not Call.   Some people attend meetings so they will feel either important or included. If you cannot identify a specific reason for attending a meeting, you should question whether to attend. If the person who calls the meeting cannot provide a good reason for your attendance, do not go.

Have Only Necessary People Attend.   Not everyone should attend every meeting. Only people who have something specific to offer, such as information, expertise, insight, or experience, should attend.

Have Agendas for All Meetings.   It is not necessary to typeset and print agendas. An agenda can be merely a list of topics handwritten on a piece of paper and photocopied for distribution. This agenda provides a focal point for managing the meeting and for informing people in advance what topics will be covered. Thus the agenda should be distributed to all participants in advance of the meeting so that adequate preparations can be made.

Be Time Wise.   Start and end meetings on time. Specify exact times to be allowed for each agenda item and comply with the schedule. Schedule meetings at times when minimum interference or interruption is expected.

Identify Specific Meeting Outcomes.   What do you hope the meeting will accomplish? What specific decisions and/or actions are expected to result from the meeting? Identify these concerns at the bottom of the agenda so that when the meeting is summarized the actions will be explicit.

Use Standup Meetings.   Occasionally, brief standup meetings are more efficient than typical conference type meetings in which people settle in and expect the meeting to last a significant period of time. With a standup meeting, people expect the meeting to be brief and to the point, and people will disperse and return to their normal duties within a relatively short time period.

End the Meeting Appropriately.   Summarize any decisions or conclusions that resulted from the meeting. Review the objectives for the meeting and explain to participants how they were achieved. Clearly define any follow-up steps that you expect to result from the meeting. Assign responsibilities for accomplishing follow-up steps and ensure they are understood. Set dates for future meetings or future activities so that people can note them on their schedule immediately.

Delegating

Delegating is a beneficial time management tool for two reasons: (1) it involves other people in accomplishing the work and contributing to the overall goals and objectives of the supervisor; and (2) it helps to motivate and develop people for future responsibilities and greater contribution to the organization.

Keep Track of All Resources Available.   Know who can help and the capabilities of the different people who are available to help. Knowing about the different resources will make it easier for you to decide to use them when it is appropirate to do so.

Evaluate the Necessity of Each Task before Delegating.   Know why it is important to do the task and give this information to the person who receives the assignment. Understand the importance and convey that importance to the person asked to complete it.

Delegate Challenging as Well as Routine Tasks.   Delegating will help motivate as well as alleviate some of your time pressures. If you give subordinates responsible and meaningful work to do, they will work more productively and at a higher level of motivation. Delegating only boring, routine jobs to subordinates creates dissatisfaction, boredom, and resentment.

Delegate "results" rather than "how to." Ask subordinates to accomplish results, but allow them to work out the details of how those results should be accomplished. Let them have freedom and responsibility to accomplish the assignments you give them.

Ask subordinates to bring you solutions rather than problems. When subordinates have been delegated meaningful responsibilities, they often return with problems for the supervisor to resolve. Ask subordinates to think through potential solutions to those problems before imposing on your time. Quite often, they will solve the problem themselves.

Correspondence

No matter how hard we try to eliminate paperwork, it is a necessary evil. Letters, memorandums, reports, and other documents will always be with us. The following activities, however, will make the time we use to develop and write correspondence more efficient.

Outline before Writing.   Outlining is especially important for proposals, reports, or any type of analysis or recommendation. Organized thoughts save time. By organizing your thoughts prior to writing them on paper, you will save time in writing and rewriting the final draft.

Use form letters when appropriate. About 80 percent of the letters we write can fit a standard format. It is a great time saver to either commit these standard formats to a word processor, a memory typewriter, or a sheet of paper that is kept on file so that when the need arises for this type of letter, you can refer to the file, pull it out, and expeditiously prepare the letter.

Use Standard Paragraphs in Standard Sentences.   A number of standard paragraphs for opening correspondence, closing correspondence, and conveying certain messages can be useful. This saves having to "reinvent the wheel" each time we are writing a new letter to someone different.

Use Postcards for Repetitive Correspondence.   Postcards are simple, easy to use, and inexpensive. Preprinted postcards can save tremendous time in reporting lab results, in notifying patients of appointments, or other routine matters.

Use Dictating Equipment.   The average person speaks at a rate of 100 to 125 words per minute. Writing speed is around 25 to 30 words per minute. It is a more efficient use of time to dictate if at all possible.

Write Responses Directly on Incoming Mail.   Rather than rewrite addresses, return addresses, and create a completely new letter, answer any questions or request for information on the incoming correspondence. Photocopy your reply and send the original back to the sender with the information that person requested. This is a tremendous time and money saver if used consistently.

Set a Goal to Keep 90 Percent of Your Correspondence to One Page or Less.   Multiple-page correspondence is significantly more time-consuming to write than single-page correspondence. If your letters are brief and concise, not only is it easier for you to process them, but it is more likely that you will receive a concise and appropriate reply from the person with whom you are corresponding.

Paper Flow

No one can argue against the importance of paperwork in the health care field. Paper flow contains important information that is essential for us in doing our jobs. Documenting illnesses, treatments, and diagnoses is essential in providing health care services. However, it is also possible for us to drown in a sea of paperwork if we are not careful. The following guidelines will help health care supervisors to stay in control of the paper situation.

Handle Each Piece of Paper Only Once after Sorting. While checking the in basket, sort your incoming paper into two basic priorities. It is either important or unimportant. Organize the important stacks in order of priority and respond to them immediately. Set the unimportant correspondences aside for times when handling them will not interfere with normal work flow. Throw out mail that is unimportant. Certain mail can be discarded without even opening the letter. Avoid having a hold basket or any other file in which you allow paper to accumulate.

Have Someone Else Open and Sort Your Mail. If possible, have a person from the clerical staff or a receptionist open and sort your mail. Have them throw away "junk mail" and prepare a preliminary prioritization of important correspondence. Perhaps that person can answer certain items without needing your input or permission.

Designate a Space in Your Desk for Working Files. Do not allow working files to accumulate on your desk. File them in an orderly manner so that they can be found easily and replaced in their proper place after you work on them.

Place Low-priority Items out of the Way. Certain requests for information or certain letters will not benefit from your action. These same items often will not suffer if you fail to act on them. Thus put them aside and refer to them only if someone follows up or makes a follow-up request.

Reading

Because our society is rapidly moving toward an information base, reading is becoming a more essential part of everyone's primary job responsibility. In the health field, we must read to stay current with the latest practices and techniques that are being devised, to keep abreast of current legislative changes in the laws and regulations that govern the field, and to acquire the information we need to do our jobs. Therefore, reading efficiently as well as effectively will become more critical as this transition toward an information society continues.

Designate Space away from or in Your Desk for Reading Material. Save all reading material until you have an opportune time to browse through it. Take it with you to peruse while waiting for a meeting to begin or while waiting in a reception area for an appointment. Use reading activity as fill-in time. Another good time for reading is during the evening as a part of relaxation. Take some reading materials home with you and find time to read while away from work.

Avoid Holding Reading Material for More than Two Weeks. If you have not read it in two weeks, it is probably not that important. However, important material should be read within that time period. If you are not able to complete your reading within two weeks of receiving materials, then allocate more time for this activity.

Review Tables of Contents and Read Only Chapters or Articles of Specific Interest. Read books and magazines the way you read newspapers. Spend time reading only items that attract your interest or attention. Do not read magazines and books on a page-by-page basis. Read only the information that is relevant to your current interests and problems.

Read bits of articles or portions of chapters before deciding to read the entire article or book. Many people waste their time reading an entire article or book before deciding it was not meaningful to them. By sampling the material first and then making a decision, you can save time.

Procrastination

Putting things off or delaying them until a later time is one major affliction of inefficient supervisors. Because of the reactive nature of the health care field, it is particularly easy to procrastinate in most health care organizations. We can always rationalize that an emergency or some other, more urgent and pressing need took priority. The following guidelines will help you to eliminate procrastination from your supervisory style.

Make Minor Decisions Quickly. Some decisions benefit from thorough analysis and from more detailed data gathering, but most do not. For those that do not, be decisive. Act quickly and move on. Do not let minor decisions pile up and become an overpowering burden. It is much easier to make a decision about them and then move ahead.

Avoid Waiting until the Last Minute. Start tasks as soon as possible. Encourage others to start quickly rather than waiting until their deadlines. Avoid the use of deadlines as much as possible because they encourage "deadline mentality." Instead, encourage people to do things as soon as the need arises and in accordance with the importance and the priority of that particular item.

Reward Yourself and Others for Completing Tasks Quickly. The more people are rewarded for task accomplishment, the more they will be encouraged to accomplish tasks on time. Rewards can be verbal recognition, a brief memorandum, a more formal letter, or some of the more tangible rewards that the organization has to offer. Most important, the reward follows task completion; thus the supervisor recognizes that the work was accomplished expeditiously.

Avoid Becoming Bogged Down on Low-value Activities. If a person is working on low-priority or low-value activities, more important activities are not being accomplished. To accomplish the most important activities, we must do them first. Always make the greatest possible effort to complete the most important work first.

Select the Best Time of Day for the Type of Work To Be Done. Some people are more mentally alert and have greater amounts of physical energy in the morning and have relatively low energy periods in the afternoon. Others are just the opposite. Determine which type of person you are and schedule your activities accordingly. Schedule independent work and creative work for the times when you are at your highest physical and mental energy levels. Schedule meetings, appointments, task forcing, and committee work when you are at relatively low energy levels. If other people are present, the work will be done. It is much easier to procrastinate when the energy is low and when you are by yourself than it is when you are in the presence of other people.

Concentrate on One Item at a Time.   Procrastination often results when too many priorities are being juggled at once. The likelihood is that the most important priorities will fall by the wayside and be delayed. To ensure that the most important priorities are accomplished, first decide which item is most important, and then concentrate on completing that task, before handling the second most important item, and so on.

Focus Attention on the Work at Hand and Avoid Preoccupation with Other Matters.   Mind wandering results in procrastination. Trying to think about a number of different issues creates confusion, a lack of clarity, lack of focus and, most important, lack of effectiveness.

Crises

Crisis management is a frustrating function in organizations, particularly in the health care field where much of the operating work is crisis-oriented. The following steps, however, can help to eliminate crisis from the workplace, even in the health care field.

Clearly Define a System for Analyzing Crises.   Different types of crises can be anticipated in advance. Not only can they be anticipated but also decision-making guidelines, policies, and standard operating procedures can be specified so that when the crises arise they can be handled in a cool, calm, and levelheaded manner. Determine which crises are likely to occur in your work area and specify guidelines for responding to the crises. Who will decide what? What information will the decision be based on? Who will be notified and who will be responsible for implementing the decisions?

Avoid overreacting to crises. Many situations become crises because the initial reactions were excessive. Keep cool, wait until receiving all the information, take the minimum amount of action necessary to handle the situation, and avoid overkill.

Provide a Cooling Period.   People often assume that during a crisis they should act immediately, regardless of whether the action is justified. Without procrastinating, it is often valuable in a crisis situation to program consciously a delay time for the crisis to be handled adequately.

Recognize Crises as Opportunities.   Not all crises create total disaster. Many are accompanied by significant opportunities. Crises, and the problems associated with them, produce new information. This new information often drives new decisions about how the organization is developing, how it should be structured, or how it can better accomplish its goals. Examine crises to see which of these opportunities may exist so that their full potential can be realized.

These categories represent the most common time wasters and identify some specific techniques to cope with them. As this presentation reveals, there are ways to handle even the most difficult time wasters. Whatever time wasters you encounter, it is important that you recognize them, that you appreciate the impact they are having on your productivity, and finally, that you take appropriate steps to handle and eliminate them so that you can have the most productive possible situation in your own work environment. The results will be greater accomplishment of personal and organizational goals, as well as a more satisfying and rewarding career.

SUMMARY

As Wilson states, "nothing is easier than being busy and nothing is more difficult than being effective." There are two keys to being effective rather than busy. The first is to recognize the nature of time. It is available in fixed quantities and a steady and predictable rate—there isn't anything we can do to time to make it different. The second key is to recognize that we have a personal responsibility to ourselves to make the best use of the time that is available to us.

Thus, "time management" is itself a misleading phrase. We should think in terms of managing ourselves *in relation to time*. This means first determining what is important to us in life and using these goals as the criteria for determining how we spend our time.

REFERENCES

Lakein, A. *How to Take Control of Your Time and Your Life.* New York: New American Library, 1972.

Mackenzie, R. A. *The Time Trap: Managing Your Way Out.* New York: American Management Association, 1972.

Wilson, M. W. *Tools and Techniques Checklist.* Self-published, 1982.

Chapter Ten

The Management of Change

Consider the following predictions:

- Hospital costs will continue to increase.
- Demand will increase.
- Total payor costs will increase.
- Government regulation of hospitals will increase.
- Government will modify benefits to reduce demand.
- Business community will explore options to reduce costs.
- Competition will intensify.
- Planning/management will improve.
- Role of some hospitals will change.
- For some, nature of business will change.
- Some hospitals will cease operating.

These predictions were made at a workshop for nurses presented by the American Hospital Association in 1984. The theme of the workshop was the new payment environment resulting from changes in the way Medicare reimbursement will be handled. In the past, Medicare reimbursed hospitals according to reasonable costs incurred in providing services. Payment was after the fact. Through the new reimbursement system, however, hospitals will be paid on a prospective basis and limits will be established on how much a hospital receives for various categories of illness and hospitalization.

Further consider the *new vocabulary* resulting primarily from changes in the reimbursement system:

- DRG (diagnosis related groups)
- CMI (case mix index)

- HCFA (Health Care Financing Administration)
- PPS (prospective payment system)
- UCR (usual, customary, and reasonable)
- RIM (relative intensive measures)

Reflect on what the following authors have said recently about the changes in reimbursement policies:

That the changes involved with prospective pricing are sweeping has been emphasized again and again. (Shaffer, 1984, p. 94)

The federal government's decision to pay hospitals prospectively by diagnosis related groups (DRGs) has suddenly and substantially altered the system. . . . (Riley & Schaefers, 1983, p. 40)

The federal government's resolve to cut health care expenditures is resulting in dramatic changes in the way hospitals are reimbursed by Medicare and Medicaid. (Mannisto, 1983, p. 9)

As a result of these changes, the health care industry is facing tremendous challenges. In addition, consider changes such as the following:

- Rapidly changing technology
- Unionization and, in some cases, strikes by nurses
- Increased ownership/management of hospitals by large profit-oriented corporations

It seems that all we see are changes.

The questions frequently asked of supervisors are: "How will you respond to change? Will you view the changes as threatening to your security and thus resist the change efforts, or will you view the changes as new opportunities?" The different philosophical viewpoints are illustrated in Figure 10.1.

If you are threatened by change and think you can survive by not allowing change to take place, look at the "stagnation" portion of the curve in Figure 10.1. If you do not change things, you will be left behind because clients' needs, employee preferences, technological capabilities, governmental regulations, and the nature of competition all change in time. Conversely, the "chaos" portion of the diagram shows the situation caused by too much change. An optimal amount of change, however, is referred to as the "managed change" portion of the diagram. In other words, supervisors must manage change or change will manage them. Managed change requires a proactive rather than reactive approach. We intend in this chapter to address topics that will provide supervisors with the skills needed to manage change.

Our objectives in this chapter include the following:

- To develop a key vocabulary regarding change.
- To understand the benefits of managing change.

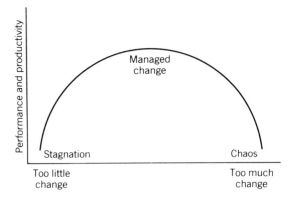

Figure 10.1. Degrees of changes.

- To understand a supervisory process for managing change.
- To understand why people resist change and how to overcome this resistance.

DEFINITION OF TERMS

The term *management of change* is defined by applying the management process to the issue of change. We define management as follows: *Management is the process of coordinating all resources through processes such as planning, organizing, controlling, and motivating to achieve desired goals and objectives.*

Furthermore, we define change as follows: *Change is the process of altering an existing state of organizational affairs to either (1) solve an existing problem or (2) avoid some future problem.*

The management of change concerns three time dimensions—past, present, and future—and produces two time perspectives about change. Let us suppose that a health clinic has not been carefully monitoring the attitudes of the staff in the clinic. During a period of time, dissatisfaction develops and turnover increases significantly. In this situation, management has a problem because of things that occurred in the past, but now you must make a decision in the present. Hence, the first perspective about change concerns issues associated with the past. In the other perspective, one must consider the future and realize that changes need to be made now (in the present) or problems will arise in the future. For example, a hospital manager who continues to operate under the "old rules", while the changes in Medicare/Medicaid described earlier are made, will inevitably have problems in the future. To avoid this problem, you should make changes in an anticipatory frame of thinking.

A related issue involves planned versus unplanned change. In some cases, the decision maker can make changes as necessary and can plan ahead regarding the entire change process. In other cases, the decision maker must react to some issue in the environment—government, competition, unions, and others—that produces an unplanned change. Assume that you decide to do something to reward your excellent employees and initiate a proposal to start an employee of the month award program. In this case, a proactive approach toward change is being followed. In another situation, however, your employer's major competitor significantly increases wages. This change by the competitor creates such pressures in your organization that wages must also be increased. This unplanned change developed in reaction to some environmental disturbance. Hopefully, you can develop a perspective toward change that is both anticipatory and planned.

Several key ideas we will discuss in this chapter are as follows:

- *Change agent*—the person who initiates change or to whom the responsibility is assigned.
- *External forces*—forces or pressure outside the organization that signal the need for change.
- *Internal forces*—forces or pressures within the organization that signal the need for change.
- *Structural change*—changing the organizational chart.
- *People-based change*—changing people's attitudes and behavior toward other people involved.
- *Technological change*—changing the type, equipment, or process that is used in delivering the product or service provided by the organization.
- *Task change*—changing the nature of the work people are performing.
- *Planned change*—change that is proactive and anticipatory in nature and pursued at the discretion of the decision maker.
- *Unplanned change*—change that is in reaction to some cause of concern.
- *Brainstorming*—a technique for obtaining ideas from a relatively small group where any and all ideas are "tossed on the table."
- *Nominal group technique*—a structured technique for obtaining ideas from a relatively small group when group members sequentially provide their ideas without discussion initially.
- *Job enrichment*—a method for changing a job by providing more autonomy, feedback, and variety.
- *Organizational development*—a planned process designed to change an organization's—in contrast to an individual's—approach toward decision making during a long-run time frame.
- *Force field analysis*—a technique for viewing resistance to change as a comparison of the driving forces behind a change and those restraining forces.
- *Unfreezing*—A part of planned change through which people realize that their old values, attitudes, and behavior are outdated or inappropriate for a particular situation.
- *Changing*—also a part of planned change that alters people's attitudes and behavior to those desired by the change agent.
- *Refreezing*—the third part of planned change in which the new ideas pursued in the changing phase become permanent.

BENEFITS OF MANAGING CHANGE

The benefits of managing change are similar to benefits received from managing any issue or resource; however, let us review a few of those applicable to the issue of change.

According to an old saying, if you do not manage change, it will manage you. This phrase reminds us of one of the first benefits. In other words, change is inevitable. To assume that any organization will experience a nonchanging environment for any period of time is naive. Therefore, a preferred behavior is to manage change actively, rather than allow it to manage you. In a related sense, the management of change allows you to avoid crisis type reactions to problems. To allow a situation to deteriorate, until a major change, an unplanned change, or a crisis response is needed, is obviously not comfortable.

A proactive, planned change style of management also benefits us by giving us immediate opportunities. Let us again use the example of changes in the Medicare/Medicaid programs. One reaction to this change could be insecurity, threat, and withdrawal. Since there have been predictions that some hospitals will cease operating because of these changes, you assume that it will happen to yours. Look at the other side of the coin, though. These changes provide the opportunity to be more efficient and deliver health care services for lower costs than the reimbursements received from the government. In essence, some people will be taking advantage of these changes and improving their situation, while others will be sitting back writing doomsday on the wall. Where will you find yourself?

A planned change perspective, therefore, will allow us to be aware of opportunities as they arise rather than having to react after they occur. Planned, managed change will also permit extensive and participative discussion before the ultimate decision has to be made. According to Naisbitt (1982), "The guiding principle of this participatory management is that people must be a part of the process of arriving at decisions that affect their lives" (p. 159). Thus, planning for change, you are allowing more time for this participation and involvement.

Change is inevitable. Although both death and taxes are inevitable, change should also be added to the list (Duncan, 1983). In fact, as illustrated in Figure 10.1, some change is preferred. The real supervisory challenge is how you will respond to change. Accept change as inevitable but remember that managed, planned change can provide opportunities.

A SUPERVISORY PROCESS FOR MANAGING CHANGE

Earlier in this chapter we said that we desire to change situations because either we have a problem or we want to make changes now to avoid future problems. Therefore, we can see that managing change and problem solving are similar. Consequently, we will use the decision-making model described earlier in this book to facilitate our discussion of a change process. You will recall that the model included the following steps:

- Define the problem
- Define objectives

- Generate alternatives
- Develop action plans
- Troubleshoot
- Communicate
- Implement

Each of these factors will be discussed in relation to managing change.

Define the Problem

From a change perspective, as stated earlier in this chapter, the problem may be caused by a situation in which present status conflicts with desired status. In this situation, resolution of the problem involves decision making to eliminate the gap between present and desired status. In other situations, the problem solving is anticipatory in nature and decisions are made now to avoid future problems.

At the strategic level, four alternatives are available (Lyles, 1982). The first strategy, called a *describe strategy,* involves providing a detailed account of the problem to trace cause and effect relationships. In the second strategy, *differentiation,* a problem is defined by comparing two situations—one that generates desired results versus the other that does not—to identify different factors in each situation. In the *reconstruction* strategy, a problem situation is recreated to isolate causes of the problem. In the last strategy, called *separation,* a larger problem is broken down into smaller ones.

All of these problem-solving strategies concern isolating the actual problem as opposed to symptoms. If changes are made that only concern symptoms and not the real problem, you will probably be faced with continuing symptoms. In other words, until your change strategy addresses the real problem, you have not effectively handled the situation.

Suppose that you notice that more employees seem to have trouble complying with the 30-minute lunch break. At first, only a few people exceeded the limit and even then on an infrequent basis. Lately, more people and even some top performers are noticed returning late from lunch. Further suppose that you say the following: "I have a problem so I will change their behavior by mildly reprimanding all future abusers." Have you handled the problem or a symptom? Perhaps the real problem is the long line in the company cafeteria and everyone is having trouble with that situation and the tardiness is not just a personal decision to be late. What we must do at this step in looking for the real problem is to ask the question, "What caused what I am observing to happen?" When you cannot trace the root of the problem back any further, you are probably close to the real problem. The question tracing may proceed similar to the following hypothetical example:

- I have noticed that morale seems to have decreased in my unit. What caused this to happen?
- It may be that our supervisors are using an inappropriate leadership style. What caused that to happen?

- We do not have a management development program nor do we even expose our supervisors to newer management ideas. What caused that to happen?
- We do not have an adequate performance appraisal system that incorporates employee growth.

We could continue with the example but the intent is to identify the underlying fundamental problem and pursue change strategies that relate to it and not just symptoms.

Another concern at this step is to consider the source of the problem. What is prompting the requirement for change? In some cases, the impetus for change may be internal to the company. Decision-making and communications processes may be breaking down. Delivery dates on ordered goods may not be being met. Morale may be low and turnover may be increasing. In other cases, the problem or necessity for change is caused by external factors. The government may require us to change our personnel practices. The competition may change, which requires us to change. Technological breakthroughs may require us to change the way our jobs are performed.

Managers and supervisors need to be sensitive to the various kinds of information received from these internal and external sources in order to handle smaller problems before they become big problems.

One last comment about problem solving—Georgia politician Bert Lance made the following statement a few years back: ''If it ain't broke, don't fix it.'' In other words, do not overreact to some minor issue as though you had a major problem.

Define Objectives

Contemplated changes should be considered in light of the organization's overall objectives. In determining objectives for changes strategies, we need to address questions such as the following:

- Where do we want to be after the changes are made?
- How much are we willing to spend or commit to solving the problem that we have identified or want to avoid?
- How much time can we allow?
- Who will be involved in the changes?

This list of questions is not meant to be all-inclusive but to be only representative of the issues involved in determining objectives. In other words, we want to establish the specifics of the what, who, when, and how of the actions that will be taken to correct (or avoid) the problem we identified in step one of the change process.

The establishment of objectives at this stage of managing change serves several purposes (Bedian & Glueck, 1983). Objectives provide guidelines for action. The objectives signal what should and should not be done. In addition, objectives function as a source of legitimacy for the undertaking of the organization's endeavors. The hospital's objective to provide medical services aimed at the detection, prevention, and cure of disease and illness provides the official sanction of the activities the hospital undertakes. Objectives also serve as benchmarks or standards against which progress can be attained. Suppose that a public health clinic determined that it had a problem with infection control because 21 incidents were reported during the past year. An objective was established to reduce the number of similar incidents to no more than eight in the upcoming year. As we move forward in time, we can use this standard of eight to evaluate whether we are making progress.

Objectives also provide a sense of motivation for employees. They become incentives and provide a target and a challenge if properly developed. Lastly, objectives provide a basis for further decision making that will occur. For example, after the objectives have been established, we can decide what we need to do in regard to organizational design, development of control measures, and so forth.

In most situations, multiple objectives must be established. If only one objective is established, we might overlook the implicit tradeoffs required in decision making and thus fail to address the multiple concerns of the overall organization. Let us assume, for example, that a hospital had a problem—excessive budget overruns. The decision makers decided to change things by mandating across the board 25 percent decreases in budget. Further suppose that the 25 percent reduction in the nursing division involved significant layoffs and patient care suffered severely. Obviously, we have traded off an undesirable event (budget overruns) for another undesirable event (poor patient care) and failed to see the "big picture." What we need then are multiple objectives that address the multiple complexities in making change. In other words, what are *all* the areas that will be impacted if a particular change strategy is pursued? Objectives need to be established for each area in which an impact will be felt.

Properly established objectives have several features (Huse, 1982).

- They form a hierarchy that is broad at the top level of the organization and more narrow and specific at lower levels of management and individual workers.
- They are well understood.
- They are balanced.
- They identify expected results.
- They consider internal and external constraints and environments.
- They are measurable and quantitative in nature.
- They are within the power of the individual responsible for their attainment.
- They are acceptable to those responsible for their attainment and others who will be affected by their attainment.

Good objectives are necessary because the decision-making process and what we ultimately decide to change will depend on the results we have identified.

Generate Alternatives

At this next step of generating alternatives, we will discuss what we can change and some techniques for involving other people in the generation of alternatives. The options that we have are as follows:

- Change people in the organization
- Change the nature of the jobs
- Change people's attitudes and beliefs
- Change the technology being used
- Change the organizational structure

In the first instance, the "players of the game" can be transferred, demoted, promoted, or rotated. Suppose that you believe the problem of decreasing morale in the unit is the management and supervisory style of the unit leader. One option—not necessarily a preferred one, but still an alternative—is to replace the present person.

Another alternative is to change the nature of the job being performed. Suppose that nurses experience frustration with the perceived fragmentation of health care when operating under the team nursing modality. Primary nursing may offer more autonomy, involvement, and continuity of care than will team nursing. In this instance, everything remains the same except that the nature of the job changes. Job design, job enrichment, job enlargement, and job rotation are ways to change the nature of the jobs being performed.

In addition, one might consider trying to change people's beliefs and attitudes on particular problems and issues. For example, a company may have traditionally discriminated against various categories of people. The discrimination was not a corporate policy as such, but became visible through managers' beliefs, attitudes, and assumptions about people. Through various intervention strategies, we can attempt to convince people to broaden their beliefs and attitudes.

The next alternative involves changing the technology. In highly technical areas, we can use more updated technology when it becomes available and if it is more cost efficient. The health care industry has known and will continue to experience tremendous changes in the technology being used. Moreover, there will be increasing pressure to adopt new, more efficient technologies because of changes in reimbursement methods by federal and state agencies.

The benefits of participatory management and decision making have been reported extensively in today's management literature. Certainly, an appropriate place for pursuing participation is when changes are being considered. When people participate in changes that are being considered, developed, and analyzed, they are more likely to be committed to the changes finally implemented. We will briefly review several techniques for generating ideas and alternatives by including the people who work in the organization.

One technique is called *brainstorming*. In brainstorming, small groups of people are formed to generate alternatives and ideas. In general four rules are followed in brainstorming (Schermerhorn, 1984).

1. All criticism of ideas is withheld until the idea generation stage is complete.
2. "Freewheeling" is encouraged. Wild, radical, and exotic ideas are welcomed.
3. Quantity of ideas is important. The more ideas generated, the more likely the superior alternatives will be discovered.
4. Combination and improvement of ideas are sought.

In brainstorming, either antagonistic arguments may develop or one or more individuals may dominate the group discussion. If such events can be predicted before the group discussion begins, an alternative technique—the nominal group technique—can be used as follows (Schermerhorn, 1984):

1. Group participants work alone and respond in writing with their own alternatives to a particular problem.
2. After adequate time has been allowed for all alternatives to be recorded, the alternatives are read aloud in a round-robin fashion, with each group member providing one alternative at a time. Successive rounds will probably be required to obtain all the alternatives.
3. As the alternatives are read, the facilitator records the alternatives on a board or chart for all group members to see.
4. The alternatives are then discussed individually. The ideas may be discussed for both clarification and evaluation.
5. A written voting procedure on the most preferred alternative(s) is followed to establish a rank ordering of the alternatives. Modifications might involve weighting of the most preferred alternative.
6. Steps 4 and 5 are repeated depending on the number of alternatives desired.

In this technique, the round robin approach ensures that everyone will have a chance to respond. The written voting procedure ensures that no one will respond because of intimidations, threat, or group pressures.

One last formal group technique that we will discuss is the quality control circle (QCC). According to Boone and Kurtz (1984), "Quality circles are volunteer groups of operative employees who periodically brainstorm on how to increase the firm's output, improve quality, or improve the efficiency of the work place" (p. 498).

In addition, according to Barra (1983), "Achieving maximum quality and productivity gains will require a change process that gradually involves more and more employees and managers in joint problem-solving and decision-making activities. . . . A change process that will create this environment is the quality circle process" (p. 46).

Develop Action Plans

Developing action plans begins after all alternatives have been generated and ends with choosing one alternative, at least tentatively. Essentially, alternatives are compared and evaluated so that managerial judgment can be applied to choosing the best available alternative. We will discuss several methods through which alternatives can be evaluated.

In the change process we are describing, we define the problem, determine objectives, and generate and evaluate alternatives, before making a choice. As we evaluate and compare alternatives, we need to remember the problem and objectives. Unfortunately, some managers will jump to a choice that does not adequately address either the real problem or the desired objectives.

Furthermore, in this evaluation stage, all costs and benefits of each alternative should be identified. Suppose, for example, you are considering two benefit plans for the employees in the hospital. Alternative one is a "lean" plan, which does not provide many extras. Alternative two has far more benefits and obviously costs more. This point is reflected in Figure 10.2 with the line labeled "strict costs of benefits package." It may be tempting to choose alternative one because, on this criterion alone, it appears to be less costly. However, the "total costs" include those behavioral and human costs involved when dissatisfied employees leave often or are absent more often than satisfied ones. One must assume that a more extensive benefits package would provide higher satisfaction and, in turn, less costs due to absenteeism and turnover. This relationship can be seen in Figure 10.2 in the line labeled "behavioral and human costs." What is important are the "total costs". Some middle ground perspective is required to handle the tradeoffs associated with competing alternatives.

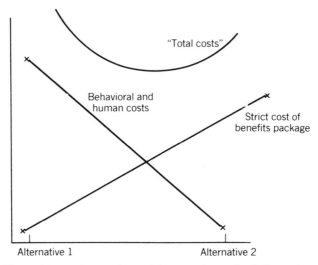

Figure 10.2. Comparison of the "total costs" of alternatives.

	Alternatives				Total
	1	2	3	4	
Alternative 1	1	2	1	4	1
Alternative 2	X	1	2	2	3
Alternative 3	X	X	1	4	0
Alternative 4	X	X	X	X	1

Figure 10.3. Comparison technique for evaluating alternatives.

Several techniques are available for making comparisons among alternatives. We will cover comparison techniques, force field analysis, and judgmental processes. Obviously, other techniques are also available.

One simple way to evaluate alternatives is to compare each alternative to the others. Suppose, for example, that you have interviewed four people for an opening in your unit. These four alternatives are listed on both edges of a lined box, as indicated in Figure 10.3. The process involves comparing each alternative to the remaining ones and deciding which is preferred. For example, when alternative one was compared to alternative two, alternative two was preferred, and a "2" was placed in that box. When alternative one was compared to alternative three, alternative one was preferred and a "1" was placed in that box. The "X" boxes show that there is no reason to compare an alternative with itself, and the comparisons below the diagonal would merely repeat those above the line. After all comparisons have been made, a count is made of the number of times each alternative is preferred and then entered in the total column. In this example, alternative two is the most preferred. Numerous extensions involve multiple criteria, and weighting methods can be added to this basic technique.

Force field analysis is a formal method for listing the pros and cons of the various alternatives being considered. Suppose, for example, your hospital's cafeteria needs major renovation. One alternative would be to close the cafeteria for three months; another might be to have patient meals catered; and a third would be to serve prepackaged, convenience foods. Let us assume that you are evaluating the alternative of whether to close the cafeteria. Table 10.1 shows some of the "forces" acting in favor of and those opposing such an alternative.

The last approach, called a *judgmental* one, is basically a philosophy of evaluation, rather than a technique. Alternatives are carefully considered usually by a group to gain the "two heads are better than one" advantage. Several rules to follow in using subjective evaluation are as follows (Lyles, 1982):

- Actively consider all alternatives.
- Actively consider all criteria.

Table 10.1

Alternative: Close Hospital Cafeteria for Three Months and Renovate

Advantages		Disadvantages
Lower price from contractor	→	
		← Patients and staff will complain because of no place to eat.
"Go ahead and finish it."	→	
		← Image of hospital may suffer.
Less likelihood of accident with customers being around construction since area will be shut off.	→	
		← May lose patients because competition is strong.
Can go ahead and do complete job.	→	
		← May take longer than three months, which makes it even worse.

- View differences of opinion as helpful.
- Avoid arguing just to win the argument.
- Do not agree just to be agreeable.
- Do not take numerical short cuts.
- Encourage everyone to participate.

As a final part of this change process, an action plan covering the who, what, when, and where issues should be developed to support the choice that has been made.

Troubleshoot

Troubleshoot should include as broad an area as possible. In other words, a decision was made but has not yet been communicated and implemented, so we have one last chance to reflect on the alternative that has been chosen. We need to ensure that this alternative is likely to change or avoid the problematical situation that exists. We might decide to have a new group review the chosen alternative to see if any issues have been overlooked. If possible, we might want to conduct a field test or simulate the change before we "do it for real." We may also do some "what if" type analysis at this stage. In the earlier example regarding the closing of the cafeteria, you might ask, "What if the renovation has been completed in three months?" Although some issues may have been considered during the examination of the alternatives, the focus here is on anticipation of future events.

Communicate

Managerial communications involve a two-way process because manager sends out a message and the recipient either does or does not respond. Thus the communications are not complete until the desired response has been observed. Suppose, for example, hospital employees have been parking in areas designated for visitors only. You decide to handle this situation by sending a memo to all department heads and asking them to either post it or discuss it with employees. You continue to receive reports that employees are not complying with the request. Managerially speaking, communications have not occurred, even though you sent a message.

In a specific sense, to communicate the intended change means writing it down or explaining it to someone. One concern that should be anticipated is negative reaction to change. People naturally resist change even though the situation may be better after the change. People resist change for several reasons (Bedian & Glueck, 1983). A person's "parochial self-interest" will cause change to be resisted. If a person believes that something of value will be lost during or after the change, it will be resisted. If people either do not understand the nature of the change or do not trust the initiators of change, resistance will occur. A different assessment of or perspective toward the proposed change will also cause resistance. Finally, some people have a low tolerance for change.

Implement

Several points must be addressed at this final step of our change process model. Two factors—timing and scope—must be specified (Ivancevich et al., 1983). Timing refers to the proper time to initiate the change action. Some hospitals are cutting back on staff in reaction to the changes caused by the new Medicare and Medicaid reimbursement method. One must consider the "when" of implementing such a change. Obviously, the time chosen for implementation should be as least disruptive as possible. The scope factor refers to the extent to which the change is introduced throughout the organization. Suppose, for example, that you are planning to implement some new technical processes in the hospital. You may elect to implement the change at once and have the hospital convert at the same time or use a phased-in approach.

Moreover, while implementation is being pursued, be sensitive to feedback (such as, "Did the problem go away?"). In other words, change is implemented only to correct or avoid some problem situation. Did the implemented change move you toward the desired position?

In addition, any change will probably have "bugs" that must be worked out. Supervisors should be prepared for probable downturns in performance as people adjust to the changes. According to Besse (1957), ten conditions exist under which the implementation of change will be more acceptable:

1. If it is understood
2. If it does not threaten security
3. If those affected have been involved
4. If it is a result of impersonal principles, rather than a personally dictated order

5. If it follows a series of successful changes rather than a series of failures
6. If the change is introduced after prior change has been assimilated
7. If it has been planned
8. If people are relatively new on the job
9. If people will share in the benefits of the change
10. If the organization expects improvements rather than static procedures

SUMMARY

Due to technological changes, revisions of government rules and regulations, and the increased demand for health care services, the medical care sector of our economy is presently facing significant changes. The following guidelines should facilitate the management of change in this environment.

- The health care industry is experiencing tremendous changes and will continue to do so.
- A supervisor must either manage change or be managed by it.
- Some degree of change is desired and beneficial.
- Change can be seen as an opportunity rather than a threat.
- Change is undertaken to either solve an existing problem or avoid some future one.
- Planned change is usually more beneficial than unplanned change.
- A participative leadership style is highly appropriate in many change situations.
- The following process can be used for managing change:
  - Define the problem
  - Define objectives
  - Generate alternatives
  - Develop action plans
  - Troubleshoot
  - Communicate
  - Implement
- We should focus on the actual problem and not just symptoms.
- The following are change options:
  - Change the people
  - Change the nature of the job
  - Change people's attitudes and beliefs
  - Change the technology being used
  - Change the organizational structure

- Brainstorming, the nominal group technique, and quality control circles are techniques for generating alternatives.
- Think about the tradeoffs involved while considering a particular change.
- People do naturally resist change, but there are ways to overcome resistance.
- Determine the timing and scope of the proposed change.

REFERENCES

Barra, R. *Putting Quality Circles to Work.* New York: McGraw-Hill, 1983.

Bedian, A. G., & Glueck, W. F. *Management.* New York: Dryden Press, 1983.

Besse, R. (1957, April). "Company planning must be planned." *Dun's Review and Modern Industry, 69,* 6203.

Boone, L. E., & Kurtz, D. L. *Principles of Management.* New York: Random House, 1984.

Duncan, W. J. *Management: Progressive Responsibility in Administration.* New York: Random House, 1983.

Huse, E. F. *Management.* St. Paul: West, 1982.

Ivancevich, J. M., Donnelly, J. H., Jr., & Gibson, J. L. *Managing for Performance.* Plano, TX: Business Publications, 1983.

Lyles, R. I. *Practical Management Problem Solving and Decision Making.* New York: Van Nostrand Reinhold, 1982.

Mannisto, M. (1983, March 16). "Managers wanted." *Hospitals, 57* (6), 91.

Naisbitt, J. *Megatrends.* New York: Warner, 1982.

Riley, W., and Schaefers, V. (1983; December). "Costing nursing services." *Nursing Management, 14*(12), 40.

Shaffer, F. A. (1984; February). "Nursing: Gearing up for DRG's part II: Management strategies." *Nursing and Health Care,* 94.

Schermerhorn, J. R. *Management for Productivity.* New York: Wiley, 1984.

Chapter Eleven

Conflict Management

Some degree of conflict is inevitable. Whenever two or more people with different values, drives, perspectives, or interests interact, a potential conflict situation exists. The term *conflict* has traditionally had negative connotations, because conflict often leads to negative outcomes. This chapter, however, discusses positive aspects of conflict and the role of supervisors in managing conflict so that positive outcomes will be realized. One study showed that the average manager spends approximately 20 percent of available time dealing with conflicts (Thomas & Schmidt, 1976). since such a significant percentage of time affects this issue, supervisors should consider this time to be an investment in making things better rather than just an expenditure of time to alleviate the conflict.

The proper assessment of this viewpoint toward conflict can be seen in Figure 11.1. In the region described by the number one, we have an undesired conflict situation. As the diagram shows, too little conflict exists. No new initiatives are being implemented. No new ideas are causing departments to respond. Stagnation and a lack of innovation lead to poor performance from both the individual and the organization. In the area described by number two, there is too much conflict, and again we have an undesired performance level. In this situation, the high degree of conflict causes chaos, which means that performance is not at the desired level. In the third situation, we are managing conflict. There is enough conflict to keep new ideas flowing, but the high degrees of conflict are avoided.

Admittedly, it will be difficult to know precisely where this level is. Some individuals and organizations can tolerate substantial conflict, while others become uneasy at the first sign of conflict. Nevertheless, positive results can be received if conflicts are managed effectively. According to Robbins (1984):

> Managers should stimulate conflict to achieve the full benefits from its functional properties, yet reduce its level when it becomes a disruptive force. But since we have yet to design a sophisticated meaning instrument for assessing whether a given conflict level is functional or dysfunctional, it remains for managers to make intelligent judgments concerning whether conflict levels in their units are optimal, too high, or too low. (p. 397)

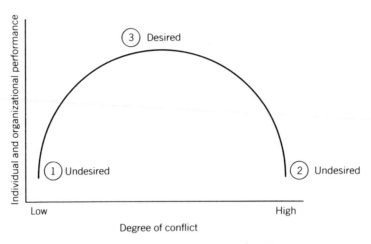

Figure 11.1.   Viewpoints toward conflict.

DEFINITION OF KEY TERMS

Conflict has been defined in several ways. The following definitions are representative examples:

> When we use the term conflict, we are referring to perceived incompatible differences resulting in some form of interference or opposition. (Robbins, 1984, p. 394)

> Conflict occurs whenever disagreements exist in a social situation over issues of substance and/or emotional antagonisms. (Schermerhorn, 1984, p. 560)

> Conflict refers to all kinds of opposition or antagonistic interaction. It is based on scarcity of power, resources and social position, and differing value structures. (Robbins, 1974, p. 23)

> Conflict might be defined as a disagreement between two or more individuals or groups. (Griffin, 1984, p. 309)

> Conflict occurs when two or more people or groups perceive that they have incompatible goals and an interdependence of activity. (Flippo & Munsinger, 1982, p. 394)

These definitions address the multiple aspects of conflict in the organizational setting. The word "perception" appeared in several of the definitions. Here the issue is not whether the differences or disagreements are real. The issue is the perception by the parties in conflict.

Another aspect of conflict is the multiple types of conflict (Schermerhorn, 1984). There can be conflict within an individual: for example, a nurse working in a clinic that decides to start offering the service of abortion may experience a conflict between personal and work values. Another type of conflict is between individuals: for example, a nurse who is in conflict with a physician may avoid going on rounds with him. Another form of conflict is between groups in a particular organization: for example, a patient's lab work may not be completed as soon as the doctor would like it. The last category of conflict occurs between organizations. There can also be conflicts between governmental agencies, unions, or insurance companies and organizations that deliver health care.

Eight different kinds of conflict that nurses might face in health care settings have been identified by Kramer and Schmalenberg (1976). The first category, called the *professional-bureaucratic conflict,* develops from the difference between the professional level of work that a nurse studies in school and the organizationally required work that a nurse performs. For example, one nurse said:

"I think the things that are most dissatisfying are the days when you are really busy, short of staff, have several critical patients, and the supervisor comes up and wants to know why the report isn't in yet or why your bathtub or utility room isn't clean yet." (Kramer & Schmalenberg, 1976, p. 21)

In the second area of conflict, called the *means-goals,* the nurse tries everything possible (uses all available means), but still experiences an undesired outcome (fails to achieve a goal): for example, when a terminally ill patient requests help but there are no means available to the nurse. In a related type of conflict, called the *personal competency gap,* the nurse lacks the necessary skills and abilities, which in turn, causes the nurse to be unable to meet personal expectations.

Three related types of conflict derive from "differential self-other role expectations." Doctor–nurse, patient–nurse, and nurse–nurse are the subcategories here. The conflict arises because of "difference in the individuals' conceptions of appropriate role behavior." In these three situations, each individual performs opposite the other individual. How these "others" perform can affect the other party and can produce conflict.

The seventh type of conflict, called the *expressive-instrumental* category, develops when the nurse is torn between the general requirement for providing health care to a number of patients and the particular needs of one specific patient. An example should clarify this category:

"I had a patient who was really worried about having a breast biopsy and she had finally opened up and was talking about it. But then it was time—in fact it was way past time—for me to pass my 6:00 P.M. meds and I didn't know if I should stay with her or pass the meds to the rest of the patients." (Kramer & Schmalenberg, 1976, p. 23)

The eighth category of conflict concerns the competing roles a nurse is required to fulfill. An individual performs as a nurse, but is also perhaps a parent, a spouse, or fiancee, and situations of conflict can arise when these roles interfere.

Several important terms that will be used in this chapter include the following:

- *Avoidance*—a conflict management strategy that attempts to bypass the problem.
- *Traditional conflict management*—a philosophy of conflict management that assumes all conflict is bad and should be removed.
- *Behavioral conflict management*—a philosophy of conflict management that assumes conflict is inevitable because "people are people."
- *Proactive conflict management*—a modern-day philosophy that assumes conflict can be good or bad and the issue becomes one of managing conflict.
- *Constructive conflict resolution*—a strategy for resolving conflict that is good for the individuals and/or organizations.
- *Destructive conflict resolution*—a strategy for resolving conflict that is harmful to the individuals and/or organization.
- *Smoothing*—a conflict management style of "patching things up" or "smoothing things over" to try and maintain harmony.
- *Win-lose conflict*—a situation in which one party to the conflict wins and the other(s) loses.
- *Lose-lose conflict*—a situation in which the multiple parties to the conflict all lose.
- *Win-win conflict*—a situation in which all parties in a conflict situation win.
- *Conflict trigger*—a force or situation that causes the likelihood of conflict to be higher than would otherwise be the case.
- *Dominance*—a conflict resolution strategy that involves forcing or imposing a solution to a conflict situation on the affected parties.

BENEFITS OF MANAGING CONFLICT

The supervisory and organizational benefits of managing conflict are numerous. At a general level, we can see the benefits in Figure 11.1. The benefits are associated with avoiding the undesirable or destructive situations (positions 1 and 2) and achieving the desired or constructive situations (position 3).

As we stated earlier, too little conflict can be destructive. It has been said that the bankruptcy of the Penn Central Railroad occurred primarily because the board of directors wanted to avoid conflict (Huse, 1982). Although several directors saw problems in the operation of the railroad, the desire to avoid a public confrontation with management led to poor decision making and the ultimate demise of the railroad.

Imagine yourself as a supervisor of nurses in a large hospital. The use of the term "supervisor of nurses" is often used in general to represent any level in the nursing hierarchy in which nursing supervision occurs. You have just recently been promoted into this job. You have some anxieties because you want to remain well liked by those nurses with whom you work. In other words, before the promotion, you were "one of them" and now you are "in charge." One day, while making rounds, you notice a newly hired nurse performing a procedure not in accordance with hospital policy. The improper procedure is neither illegal nor life-endangering. You decide not to confront the nurse because to do so might generate conflict between you and the nurse. Eventually, however, this nurse becomes more careless in the procedures being used, and finally, the use of an improper procedure leads to complications during recovery, an upset patient, and a lawsuit. Trying to avoid conflict merely created a negative situation. Earlier attention to this situation, even though it might have produced some conflict, would have resulted in long-run improvements. This example represents a situation at position one in Figure 11.1. Benefits would have been received by moving from position one to two.

To illustrate the other situation of too much conflict leading to negative outcomes, consider the following situation. Two hospitals reached an agreement in which one, having its own ambulance service, would also deliver patients to the other hospital. Sharing one ambulance service would result in higher levels of efficiency. After a period of smooth operations, however, some conflict begins to develop. The hospital that does not have the ambulance service believes that the other hospital is not servicing it fairly. Attempts at reaching some solution are not successful, and the shared arrangement is terminated. Now both hospitals have their own separate ambulance services, and the community suffers because costs increase since neither hospital alone is realistically able to support a separate ambulance service.

Another way to examine the benefits of managing conflict can be seen in win-win, win-lose, and lose-lose strategies. In a win-win strategy, both parties to a dispute or conflict situation win. Suppose, for example, that the hospital cafeteria lines become quite long during the serving hours. Staff, visitors, and patients complain about the excessive wait in the line. Cafeteria personnel complain about the unevenness in the workloads. At times, there is little to do, but at other times near chaos prevails. A possible solution might be to schedule the hours of operation so that staff members eat the noonday meal from 11 A.M. to 12 P.M., and patients and visitors eat from 11:30 A.M. to 12:30 P.M. This solution provides 30 minutes of time for staff, 30 minutes of overlap, and 30 minutes for visitors and patients. Agreeing with the feasibility of the proposed solution is less important than identifying the potential for a win-win situation. Because the lines are more manageable, the staff, visitors, and patients do not complain, and the cafeteria workers respond favorably to a more uniform flow of people.

In a win-lose strategy, one party to the conflict gains and the other loses. Suppose, for example, you supervise two people who have a serious personality clash. You have tried different ways to eliminate or reduce the conflict and nothing seems to work. You finally decide to separate the two people by placing each person on a different shift. They both prefer the present shift and you decide to use reverse seniority as the criterion for moving the junior person to an undesired shift. The senior person ''wins'' because the personal conflict is removed and the desired shift of work is retained. The junior person ''loses'' because the work shift is not preferred. Furthermore, you, as the supervisor, may ''lose'' because the dissatisfied junior person might react with an increase in absenteeism, decrease in morale, or even resignation.

The third category is the lose-lose situation. Assume, in the example just described, the two people have reached such a state of conflict that they have an open, hostile, physical confrontation in a patient's room. You try to resolve the conflict by saying "nice people don't fight", and everyone is a loser. The real problem remains but the patient, the two people, the remaining staff members, you, and the organization have "lost".

In considering these three examples, try to avoid the lose-lose and win-lose situations and pursue the win-win combinations. While ideally a win-win strategy is preferable, some situations may provide for only a win-lose response. Such a situation would still be preferable to a lose-lose one.

A SUPERVISORY PERSPECTIVE TOWARD CONFLICT MANAGEMENT

Because views toward conflict management have changed, a supervisor should use the most current and relevant perspective for effective managerial decision making. The three views that have emerged are called traditional, behavioral, and interactionist (Robbins, 1984).

The traditional viewpoint, prevalent in the early part of this century, assumed that conflict was always bad and destructive. The supervisor's job was to eliminate conflict. This philosophy would imply a top-down approach to conflict resolution.

Through 1940 to 1970, the behavioral view became popular. This viewpoint accepted conflict as inevitable. In other words, the "people will be people" attitude meant that any time two or more people interacted, conflict would occur. Conflict, however, was not always seen as bad.

In the modern era, the interactionist viewpoint recognizes that conflict can be either good or bad depending on how it is managed. A supervisor with the interactionist attitude encourages conflict if there is not enough to generate action. This approach certainly differs from the behavioral one, which merely accepted conflict. An interactionist takes a proactive role and stimulates conflict if it is observed to be at unacceptably low levels. Furthermore, as indicated earlier, an interactionist viewpoint realizes that both constructive and destructive outcomes exist in conflict situations.

The resolution strategies under these three philosophies are shown in Table 11.1. The two major distinctions of the interactionsist philosophy are (1) at times conflict will have to be stimulated and (2) conflict can be either good or bad depending on how it is managed. It is important for a supervisor to incorporate these two features

Table 11.1
Differing Views On and Solutions To Conflict

Traditional	"Stop your bickering and go back to work."
Behavioral	"Come on now; can't we all compromise a little?"
Interactionist	"What's the *real* problem here?"

into the development of a personal managerial philosophy. According to Kramer and Schmalenberg (1976):

> Conflict can be health and growth producing if it is managed constructively. Nursing is rich with conflicts. If these were resolved constructively we would see an improvement in patient care and increased job satisfaction for the nurse. (p. 25)

WHAT CAUSES CONFLICT

Earlier we described various types of conflict, and here we will describe the various causes of conflict. Although many causes of conflict exist, we developed our list from works by Huse (1982) and Robbin (1974, 1984).

The first category results from two or more organizational units having conflicting goals. In an earlier chapter, we described the situation that now exists because of changes in Medicare and Medicaid reimbursement procedures. One part of the change establishes limits for various types of patient care and the provider of service will receive only a flat fee regardless of how long the patient stays. Let us assume in a hypothetical case that a patient has been admitted to a hospital for a certain service that has a five-day standard for time of stay. In other words, the hospital will be paid for only five days of stay, regardless of whether fewer or more days were actually required. Further assume that the hospital is facing a revenue crunch. Perhaps a hospital official, who is overly concerned about costs, might try to send these hypothetical patients home early or allow them to stay only five days. The viewpoint is, "We will lose money if these patients stay any longer." Someone in the hospital, who is more concerned about patient care, might say: "I don't care how long it takes, this patient needs additional care." Hopefully, this exaggerated example will not happen, even though such predictions have been made. In another, perhaps more realistic example, physicians often want the latest in equipment and technology in the hospitals where they practice. A person, who is concerned about finances and has goals different from the physician's, may view the situation differently and prefer acceptable and not elaborate equipment. Different perspectives, goals, or interests produce potential conflict.

Our second source of conflict results from work activities among various individuals or units that are dependent on or interrelated to one another. Nursing activities are dependent on those for which housekeeping is responsible. If one or the other does not perform as expected, conflict can result. This type of conflict can be prevalent in hospitals where 24-hour service is provided and typically three shifts are used. What one person does or does not do on one shift affects what the next shift does or cannot do. If activities are not completed as required on one shift, there can be conflict when the next shift has to do, undo, or redo the earlier shift's work.

Scarce resources also provide a source of conflict. There are never enough monetary resources to accommodate all requests. This source of conflict is illustrated by the "there's only so much to go around" philosophy. Consider, for example, the following description:

> A hospital's nursing department and radiology department may agree that improving patient care is a primary objective. But the nursing department may want to spend money on in-service training and on hiring nursing specialists, whereas the radiology department may want to purchase an expensive piece of equipment. Generally, the hospital cannot afford both. (Huse, 1982, p. 522)

The fourth source of conflict is based on communications problems. Misunderstood and/or unclear instructions, semantics, communication style, "noise" or any other barrier or interference in the communication flow can create conflict. Suppose a supervisor tells an employee: "Work on this as soon as you can." The employee interprets this as: "Work on this when you finish what you are working on now." The supervisor really meant, "Work on this right now." These different interpretations can be a source of conflict.

Individual differences in values, beliefs, interests, and attitudes can produce conflict. All of us have different backgrounds, education, work and family experiences, religious beliefs, and personalities, and these differences can create conflict. For example in one hospital, a black female nurse is being considered for promotion to a supervisory position in the nursing department. A while male physician in the hospital has such strong prejudices against blacks that he consults with the director of nursing and strongly encourages the director to appoint someone else. His value system, even though an improper one, produces conflict. This source of conflict is also a potentially strong one in health care where differences of opinion exist regarding such issues as abortions, ending the life of a terminal patient, and providing care for the indigent.

The organizational philosophy can also cause conflict with an individual's preferences. Organizations can be described in general as organic or mechanistic (Burns & Stalker, 1961). Mechanistic organizations are the classical type that use rules, procedures, decision making, and a formal hierarchical environment to accomplish the job. Organic organizations are more open and dynamic and are concerned more with the objectives to be achieved than with the particular regimen that is followed. Suppose, for example, a person has a low tolerance for rules, prefers to be allowed to make important decision, and wants general rather than strict supervision. A mechanistic structure that relies on rules, procedures, chain-of-command, and formal authority would not provide such policies. Obviously a conflict could arise.

In Chapter 10, we described the significant changes occurring in the field of health care. Consider, for example, the following advice on how organizations should be structured in certain or uncertain environments:

> Organizations or units existing in a relatively certain environment with a stable technology are best organized along bureaucratic lines with clear chains of command and specific rules and regulations; that is, they should have a mechanistic structure. Those existing in an uncertain environment with quickly changing technology are best designed along relatively open lines; that is, they should have an organic structure. (Huse, 1982, p. 523)

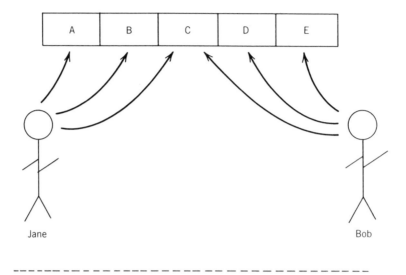

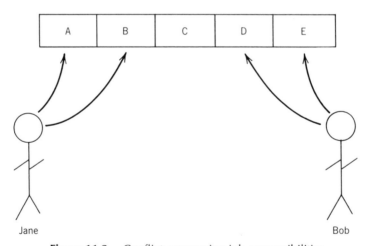

Figure 11.2.   Conflict concerning job responsibilities.

The environment that health care is facing is relatively uncertain due to the changes taking place in procedures and medical technology. In other words, the advice is the following: *Health care organizations should be organized along organic lines to avoid excessive conflict and to survive in a rapidly changing environment.*

The seventh area of potential conflict develops from overlapping or ambiguous job responsibilities. This situation can be illustrated in Figure 11.2. Assume, for example, five jobs or areas of responsibility exist in a particular unit. We will refer to these items as activities A, B, C, D, and E. Let us say those five activities are the responsibility of Jane and Bob. As can be seen in the upper part of Figure 11.2, Jane

is definitely responsible for activities A and B, while Bob is responsible for activities D and E. The conflict arises concerning activity C. Because of some uncertainty, both feel that activity C is their responsibility. Such a situation might arise
from overlapping job descriptions. The lower part of Figure 11.2 shows another
type of conflict because of an unclear situation regarding activity C. Jane is definitely responsible for activities A and B, while Bob is responsible for activities D and
E. No one has been assigned the responsibility for activity C, and conflict will
probably arise when someone realizes that this area of responsibility is not being
carried out. In this case, incomplete job descriptions or lack of clarity regarding
responsibilities could produce the situation.

The eighth source of conflict is time and priority pressures. Having more work
than available time or having conflicing or uncertain priorities regarding multiple
tasks can produce stress and conflict. Deadlines represent a specific type of pressure
device. As suggested throughout this chapter, conflict can be either destructive or
constructive. A deadline, if realistic, can be constructive and can trigger added
performance. If the deadline is unrealistic, however, the person will probably feel
overwhelmed and tend to give up.

Unreasonable standards, rules, and procedures can also cause personal and organizational conflict. If a person feels frustrated, insulted, or stymied by excessive
administrative requirements, not only does conflict arise but performance is also
negatively affected. We earlier described a state-level health care department in
which all employees were required to sign in and out when taking their 15-minute
breaks in the morning. The staff considered this procedure not only insulting because of the implied lack of trust but also a useless device for trying to maintain
control. The bitter irony is that not only did conflict arise, but it also reached such a
level that far more time was lost because people complained about the procedure to
one another and to their supervisors.

The last source of conflict is based on status differentials. We do things in
organizations that send the signal that one category of employees—those higher up
in the organizational hierarchy—is a better class of people than those lower in the
hierarchy. How many of the following examples have you seen?

- Reserved dining rooms for doctors in hospitals
- Reserved parking places for senior executives
- Lower-level employees punch time clocks, while managers do not
- Rest rooms reserved for ''special'' categories of people

To the extent that such differentials serve some meaningful purpose, they can be
defended. In many cases, though, these devices are merely status symbols and
create resentment, frustration, and conflict among those not receiving the benefits.

If we better understand what causes conflict, we should be more prepared to
recognize and manage conflict when it occurs. While other sources of conflict
probably exist, these ten areas represent the major types of conflict that will be
encountered.

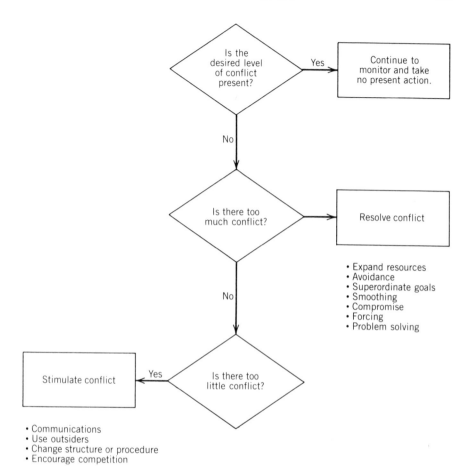

Figure 11.3. Conflict management model.

HOW SUPERVISORS MANAGE CONFLICT

We have emphasized throughout this chapter that conflict management has two separate dimensions. We have traditionally viewed conflict management in terms of conflict resolution. As we have seen in this chapter, sometimes a supervisor has to stimulate conflict. Too much conflict needs resolution, and too little conflict needs stimulation.

Figure 11.3 provides an overview of a supervisory conflict management model. One possibility is that the supervisor has been effectively managing the situation, and conflict is in control. The second possibility is that too much conflict exists, and several resolution strategies are indicated in Figure 11.3. The third possibility, and only realized recently, is that not enough conflict exists, and several stimulation strategies are also indicated in Figure 11.3. We will now explain in further detail the various strategies.

HOW TO RESOLVE CONFLICT

We will present seven methods through which a supervisor can resolve conflict. These methods are further discussed in books by Robbins (1974, 1984) and Huse (1982). Obviously, combination strategies can be invoked and our listing implies no prioritization nor likelihood of success. Under the right set of circumstances, any one of these strategies will work and under the wrong set of circumstances, none will work. It can be stated that genuine problem-solving strategies are probably preferred.

Expansion of Resources

Suppose that the housekeeping department and the physical plant department in a hospital have each asked for an additional office to house a newly employed supervisor. Also assume that only one office is available. The stage is set for conflict, but if the resource base of offices can be expanded, the conflict concerning who receives the office can be eliminated. Although such a strategy is possible, the usual implication is that added monetary resources are involved or that a tradeoff situation, which indirectly involves costs, exists. For example, we might gain an office by converting a former storeroom, but an opportunity cost may be associated with the lost storage space. At times, monetary or other restrictions mean that this strategy is not always available.

Avoidance

The avoidance approach to conflict resolution is to ignore the situation and hope it will go away. Although this technique is commonly used, it tends to be a short-run, stalling approach that does not resolve the underlying sources of conflict.

Occasionally, the avoidance technique is acceptable. Two people working in your unit, for example, clash at work because of some source of conflict. The confrontation might be work-related, personal in nature, or nonwork related. If, in your judgment, the confrontation becomes explosive primarily because each person is just having a "bad day," the avoidance strategy is likely to be more successful. By intervening when you do not need to, you may be making a "mountain out of a molehill." Conversely, the source of the conflict may have deeper roots; thus avoiding the situation only makes it worse. Extreme sensitivity and good judgment are required here because it may be difficult to distinguish between the two situations.

Superordinate goals

Superordinate goals are more important than those held by either of the conflicing parties. In this resolution strategy, we appeal to the higher set of goals as a basis for the ultimate decision. In a conflict over limited office space, for example, the conflict could become so intense that the two parties would be trying to "win" the same office space. By appealing to the higher level goal of providing proper health care, the person who manages each of the two conflicting parties can say: "If we don't start working together, patient care will suffer."

Smoothing

Smoothing is a resolution technique that involves deemphasizing differences in conflicting parties and emphasizing similarities. The resolving agent, for example, would say: "Don't worry about it. It's not that big a deal. Things will get better. We're all in this together. Let's be team players." Smoothing, however, is not an effective strategy if underlying problems are not resolved.

Compromise

A compromise strategy occurs when each party to the conflict must give up something and neither party completely wins or loses. The compromise strategy can be used when it is necessary to achieve temporary settlements to complex issues, to arrive at expedient solutions under time pressure, and as a backup when authoritative commands or problem solving are unsuccessful (Schermerhorn, 1984).

Forcing

Forcing occurs when the manager or supervisor uses the formal authority of the organizational role and mandates a resolution. In other words, the decision is "forced" on the conflicting parties. In emergency situations and in unpopular decisions such as employee cutbacks, the supervisor may have to force a solution, but in most cases, preferred alternatives are available.

Problem Solving

Though not always possible or appropriate, a genuine, united approach to solving the real problem is usually the most desirable way to resolve conflict. It does require time, but the time should be seen as an investment instead of an expenditure. By devoting time to the real problem now, you might avoid spending far more time on the problem in the future.

HOW TO STIMULATE CONFLICT

Robbins (1974) suggested that supervisors occasionally need to stimulate conflict. He stated that conflict stimulation is needed when "yes" answers are given to the following questions (Robbins, 1984):

- Has "group-think" set in so that all you see and hear are "yes" people?
- Are too many supervisors trying to be "liked" by their people rather than trying to accomplish the job?

- Is there a lack of new ideas?
- Is there an unusually low level of turnover?
- Is there too much of a sense of compromising, "smoothing over," and avoiding?

We will now review several techniques proposed by Robbins (1984) to stimulate conflict.

Communications

Two issues are associated with the use of communications to stimulate conflict. First, people must be informed that some degree of conflict is preferred. Some managers and supervisors seem to convey the idea that conflict is to be avoided so that peace and harmony can prevail. As we have already seen, managed conflict can be constructive, and this attitude needs to be fostered in the organization. Differing ideas, challenging questions, and a problem-solving attitude will result in more original, creative solutions. According to Huse (1982), "The single most effective way of stimulating manageable conflict is to let subordinates know that constructive disagreement has its legitimate place" (p. 539).

The second aspect concerns the process of communications. In other words, how communications are used can stimulate conflict and, in turn, added performance. In an earlier chapter, we described changes in the health care system that would result from changes in reimbursement mechanisms. Some people have predicted cutbacks of employees and even the closing of some health care providers. Suppose, for example, that the following memorandum is distributed in your organization:

TO: All Department Heads
Because of a severe cutback in funds, we are forced to pursue cost saving measures. Please examine the activities and operations for which you are responsible
and we will meet in ten days to discuss your ideas.

Although the message would probably contain more background information, the point is communications will stimulate new thinking and will lead to more efficient operations. Communications channels can also be used to deliver threatening or ambiguous messages (Robbins, 1984). In this sense, the threatening message might be similar to the following:

- Unless improvements are made in our operation, we will be forced to reduce the number of employees in some units.
- Some people have been abusing the sick leave policy. Unless the situation improves, we will have to consider changes in the present policy.

Ambiguous messages can also prompt recipients to seek new information and to clarify issues before they take action.

Use Outsiders

The philosophy in this conflict stimulation is to "shake things up" and receive a new perspective. The "outsider" can be someone from outside the organization or someone transferred from another department. The goal is to bring a new set of ideas, values, and outlook to a decision-making situation.

Change Organizational Structure or Procedures

Organizational units can be rearranged to stimulate new reporting relationships or alignment of areas of responsibilities. This head-to-head confrontation can be constructive if the process is managed well.

Operating procedures can also be changed to generate new points of interaction among units. Such interactions can be stimulating by moving us out of "the same old rut." For example, a state health care agency allowed operating units to develop any and all forms that might be needed in program areas. Of course, numerous inefficiencies resulted. The procedure was changed, however, to provide a clearinghouse function for all new forms, and the subsequent result was improved operations.

Encourage Competition

"The use of bonuses, incentive pay, and awards for outstanding performance are likely to stimulate competition which can lead to productive conflict as individuals and groups try to outdo each other" (Robbins, 1984, p. 403). As the competition occurs, it is likely that all or many of the competitors will rise to levels beyond what would have otherwise been the case. Numerous organizations use something similar to employee-of-the-month award. If this award includes rewards that are valued by employees, the performance of many employees will probably be stimulated along positive lines as they strive to earn the award.

SUMMARY

Supervisors should remember two important points about the process of managing conflict. Conflict can be constructive as well as destructive. The supervisory challenge is to take the lead and manage the situation to receive constructive outcomes, rather than negative ones. Second, the changed philosophy of conflict management advocates conflict stimulation. Too little conflict can be just as harmful as too much conflict.

The following items represent additional important points concerning conflict and conflict management:

- A problem-solving attitude toward conflict is preferred if time and other situational factors allow for it.

- Supervisors and managers spend a considerable amount of time resolving conflicts.
- Conflict has many sources and the more informed the supervisor is regarding these sources, the better prepared he or she will be.
- There are several methods for resolving conflict, and the supervisor will have to evaluate each situation to determine the appropriate choice.
- Some of the easier techniques for managing conflict, such as avoiding a situation or smoothing it over, will probably not resolve the real problem, and the conflict will remain or become worse.
- Three supervisory reactions to conflict can be categorized as avoiding, problem solving, and stimulation. The latter two are the preferred choices.

REFERENCES

Burns, T., & Stalker, G. M. *The Management of Innovation.* London: Tavistock, 1961.

Flippo, E. B., & Munsinger, G. M. *Management.* Boston: Allyn & Bacon, 1982.

Griffin, R. W. *Management.* Boston: Houghton Mifflin, 1984.

Huse, E. F. *Management.* St. Paul: West, 1982.

Kramer, M., & Schmalenberg, C. (1976, October). "Conflict: The cutting edge of growth." *Journal of Nursing Administration,* pp. 21–23.

Robbins, S. P. *Management: Concepts and Practices.* Englewood Cliffs, NJ: Prentice-Hall, 1984.

Robbins, S. P. *Managing Organizational Conflict: A Nontraditional Approach.* Englewood Cliffs, NJ: Prentice-Hall, 1974.

Schermerhorn, J. R. *Management for Productivity.* New York: Wiley, 1984.

Thomas, K. W., & Schmidt, W. H. (1976, June 2). "A survey of managerial interventions in respect to conflict." *Academy of Management, 19,* 315.

PART FOUR

SUPERVISION IN THE WORLD OF HEALTH CARE

Chapter Twelve

Applications of Supervisory Management Principles

Throughout the preceding chapters, we have introduced numerous supervisory management concepts and ideas. We not only expose you to these concepts, but we also encourage you to use them in your own environment. Since we can not interact with you directly, we include this chapter 15 critical incidents that are representative of problems and issues that supervisors confront. The problems and settings develop from various bases. In many cases, the incident represents a "real world" situation that we have encountered in our consulting and training.

WHAT IS A CRITICAL INCIDENT?

A critical incident is some type of disruptive situation that requires a supervisory response. Critical incidents typically represent some kind of problem or conflict that requires a supervisor to make a decision. In that sense, the incidents simulate the "real world."

HOW TO USE THE CRITICAL INCIDENTS

The following guidelines should be helpful in learning from the critical incidents.

- Do not be concerned about the organizational setting in which the incident occurs. For example, if the setting of the incident is a hospital and you work for a federal health care agency, analyze the case from a supervisory viewpoint.
- In a similar manner, do not be concerned about the functional area in which the

incident occurred. If you are a nurse and read an incident about a problem in the maintenance department, benefits still exist if you analyze the incident from a supervisory management perspective.

- Make assumptions about the incidents as long as your assumptions do not conflict with other information included.
- In considering solutions to the problems posed, try to consider the actual problems and handle them, but avoid treating symptoms.
- Do not be concerned about finding just the problem, because several problems may be present. Since management and supervision are multi-faceted, interrelated topics, the solutions prescribed will also be of the same type.
- The incidents have not been developed to reflect a chapter-by-chapter coverage nor are they presented in any particular sequence.

A NURSE'S MISTAKE

"Dispensing Wrong Drug is Common, Doctors Report" (from *The Macon Telegraph and News*, January 20, 1984)

BOSTON (AP)—Doctors who investigated a fatal mixup in which children were injected with the wrong drug say such errors in hospitals are being reported "with alarming regularity."

One newborn died and five others fell seriously ill two years ago when they were mistakenly injected with a medicine that was meant to be inhaled.

The investigators blamed the tragedy on nurses' failure to read look-alike labels. The erroneously injected inhalant was packed in a bottle that appeared identical, at a glance, to vials of vitamin E—the medicine that the youngsters were supposed to receive.

The incident at the Hospital for Sick Children in Toronto was investigated by doctors from the U.S. Center for Disease Control and the Canadian Laboratory Center for Disease Control.

The researchers said other reports show that errors occur in as many as one in six doses of medicine that are administered in hospitals.

Although most of these cause no problems for patients, they wrote, "instances of drug errors that do result in morbidity and mortality are reported with alarming regularity, as are potentially serious errors detected just before the drug is administered."

A report on the investigation of the mixup, directed by Dr. Steven L. Solomon of the U.S. Center in Atlanta, was published in today's *New England Journal of Medicine.*

"This could have happened anywhere," said Dr. William J. Martone, one of the CDC researchers. "Even when bottles are not labeled similarly, medication errors occur in hospitals. Many of the errors go unnoticed because they are inconsequential. Dosage errors may also occur."

"I can't believe that I read this in the paper after it just happened to us." Jo, the director of nursing at Fairhope General Hospital, was reading the report from the night nursing supervisor, which described a situation similar to the one in the newspaper article. A staff nurse at Fairhope had started an intravenous solution of Keflin. The doctor had prescribed ampicillin. Although complications will probably not develop, the fact remains that a mistake has been made. Because of the recent reminder in the newspaper article, Jo decides to call Barbara, the night supervisor, at home.

"Good morning, Barbara," Jo said, "I hate to bother you after you worked all night but I've just read your writeup about the Keflin and ampicillin and I would like you to do two things tonight when you come back to work," stated Jo. (Barbara was the night supervisor on whose shift the incident occurred.) "First, I would like you to talk to Sam Rogers who made the mistake and get all the facts about what happened. Then, I would like you to recommend what, if anything, we should do about Sam. I am not sure whether we should just chalk this up as a mistake or whether we should take strong action. Any questions?"

"No, I understand," replied Barbara. "I talked with Sam last night and I think it was just a mistake but I'll check into it further."

"Fine—I'll talk to you later."

After Barbara, had an opportunity to review the situation, she concluded that an honest mistake had been made. Sam had a good technical background and, according to other nurses he was quite professional at all times. He had not made a similar mistake in the past. The only contributing factor Barbara could identify was that the nurses in the unit were extremely busy and shorthanded when the improper solution was administered, and the situation may have happened because of the rush.

Barbara knows that she can adequately handle Jo's first request because she has not received any conflicting information and she feels fully informed. While waiting for Jo to arrive, however, she still has not decided how to handle Jo's second request. What, if anything, should be done with Sam?

Questions for Discussion

1. Without attempting an evaluation, list all the alternatives for handling Sam, ranging from doing nothing to immediate dismissal.

2. Which of the alternatives that you outlined seems the most appropriate? If you were Barbara, which one would you personally prefer to administer?

3. What determines the kind of action that should be used in such matters? In other words, if this had been Sam's second or third offense, would your choice of alternatives be different? If more serious complications were likely to arise, would your actions be different? In this situation, no further complications were anticipated. If the patient had an adverse reaction, would your action be different? If the patient died, would your action be different? Specifically, on what bases and at what level do you "draw the line" between a neutral, positive, or negative response as a supervisor?

THE BEST LEADERSHIP STYLE

People whose lives are affected by a decision must be a part of the process of arriving at that decision. (Naisbitt, 1982, p. 159)

The new leader is a facilitator, not an order giver. (Naisbitt, 1982, p. 188)

"Everytime I read those two sentences I say to myself '"I wish I had said that,'" Bill Smallings said to his wife, Jill, as they shared thoughts after the evening meal.

"Well, if I know you, that's my impression of how you try to manage," responded Jill. "You certainly seem to think highly of your people and they seem to respond."

"I do trust my people and try to involve them in decision making at every opportunity," agreed Bill. Bill is a supervisor of six people at University Hospital. His unit is called the Evaluation and Research Unit, and the people working with him are management analysts, operations researchers, statisticians, and planners. The unit conducts management studies designed to improve efficiency and effectiveness at the hospital. The hospital's budget is 15 million dollars and there was a growing concern that these dollars be spent wisely. "All my people are true professionals," Bill continued. "They are thinkers and doers. Because their work is so high level and technical, much of the time I don't even know what they are doing. When the statisticians start rattling off those complicated formulas, I just nod in agreement. These people would be offened if I looked over their shoulders too much, so I just outline the studies and identify available resources, and they take it from there."

"One thing is puzzling to me, though," Bill added. "While I think facilitating leadership is the best style to use, I see other people using different approaches and they seem to be successful using their own styles."

"I'll bet Jim Abrams would be one of those 'other ones'," Jill replied quickly. (Jim Abrams is a close friend of Bill's, and both families often enjoy social activities together during their leisure hours.)

Jim supervises approximately 25 people in the maintenance department at University Hospital and runs a "tight ship."

"He sure is," said Bill. "Even though he is a good friend of mine, he handles work differently. The other day we were discussing our work situations and he said that his people only worked for money. He said he had tried once or twice to involve his people in decision making but they resented it and told him that was his job. I know that most of his people have only a high school education, but I don't really think education should make that much difference. Quite frankly, one reason Jim works such long hours is that he makes all the decisions—and I do mean all. What puzzles me though is that his people seem to accept it. His absenteeism and turnover problems are no worse than anyone else's. I'd like to see his reaction if I sent him an anonymous note 'The new leader is a facilitator, not an order giver'."

"From what I've seen, you two are different kinds of people," responded Jill.

"I've noticed that when we get together he seems to treat his family the same way he treats his employees."

"Well, at least I've noticed someone in-between Jim and me. While I take a 'hands off' approach and Jim takes the 'hands on' approach, Beverly Atkins takes a 'hands joined' approach," said Bill reflectively.

"I don't know her," answered Jill, "and what do you mean by 'hands joined'?"

"I don't think you met her yet. She is the new supervisor in the business office and works right across the hall from me," replied Bill. "By 'hands joined,' I mean she joins right in and almost works right at the same level as the people who work for her. I overheard a discussion she was having with her people the other day and it was almost like they were voting on things. Everything seemed so democratic."

Later that evening, Bill reflects on the ideas of facilitating and participatory management. He knows that his own leadership style is quite compatible but he wonders how Jim and Beverly are also apparently successful when their styles are different from his. As he becomes philosophical, he imagines a leadership continuum like the one below:

Jim Abrams	Beverly Atkins	Bill Smallings
Autocrat	Consultant	Group Facilitator

Questions for Discussion

1. What do you think accounts for the apparent success of these three leaders with rather different leadership styles?
2. Do you agree with Naisbitt's statement that "people whose lives are affected by a decision must be a part of the process of arriving at that decision"? Would you use "must" if you were making a similar statement?
3. What are some of the determinants involved in deciding on a leadership style?

WHO IS IN CHARGE?

Beth Roberts recently resigned her job at County Hospital and now works as a registered nurse on a bloodmobile team for the Red Cross. Her decision to leave the hospital was not based on money; in fact, she makes less money now than she did at the hospital. Another, slightly negative aspect of the new job is the occasional overnight travel. The home office for the Red Cross is in Atlanta, and Beth's team travels the state of Georgia. About twice a month, the team stays out of Atlanta overnight in order to start early on the next day's blood drive. Despite less money and the requirement to travel, however Beth feels she has made the right decision to leave hospital nursing. A major factor prompting her decision to leave was the requirement to work rotating shifts. Beth recently had a baby and child care was extremely difficult to arrange on a rotating schedule. At least now, with predictable hours, she can make more definite arrangements for her baby.

After a couple of months on the blood team, Beth's unit has traveled to Savannah, Georgia, for a one-day drive at Armstrong State College. This trip is Beth's first to Savannah. They are having quite a turnout for the drive and events seem to be developing rather well.

On several occasions, as donors finish at Beth's station, she notices an improper procedure occurring in escorting them to the refreshment station. Mr. Stevens, an elderly volunteer, is just standing and pointing the donors to the refreshment station. On some occasions, he walks alongside the donor, but requirements specifically call for him to take the arm of the donor during the escort. Several weeks before, a donor had fainted on the way to the refreshment station and had cut her head. Beth's team is obviously somewhat sensitive to this issue.

The first few times Beth sees this situation, she says nothing to Mr. Stevens, assuming it is an oversight on his part. After noticing that Mr. Stevens routinely carries out the escort in this way, Beth decides to mention the problem to him.

"Mr. Stevens, I'm Beth Roberts. I don't believe we have met before, but we have a procedure that calls for taking the donor's arm during an escort and I notice you don't do that."

"Oh, hello, Mrs. Roberts. I haven't met you before either," replies Mr. Stevens. "This must be your first trip to Savannah."

"Yes, it is," says Beth.

"I'll try to remember what you said about the escort, Mrs. Roberts," promises Mr. Stevens. "I hope I don't forget. I've been doing this volunteer work for seven years and you know the old saying—'You can't teach an old dog new tricks'—but I'll sure try."

During the day, Beth observes that Mr. Stevens usually follows her suggestion, but on a few occasions continues to resort to his old ways.

About six weeks later, Beth's team returns to Savannah and as Beth and her team are setting up the work station, Mr. Stevens arrives.

"Good morning, Mrs. Roberts. Welcome to Savannah again," responds Mr. Stevens cheerfully.

"How are you, Mr. Stevens?" Beth inquires. "I notice on the schedule that you and I will be working together again."

"Yes, I saw that also," Mr. Stevens says. "That sounds fine to me."

For the first several donors, Mr. Stevens properly escorts the people to the refreshment stand. After an hour or so, Beth notices that Mr. Stevens is again slipping back to his old ways.

"Mr. Stevens on the last trip we talked about the importance of taking the donor's arm." Beth reminds him in a nonthreatening way.

"I told you I'd probably forget," Mr. Stevens apologizes. "I'll make sure it doesn't happen again and thanks for reminding me."

Beth notices that Mr. Stevens follows the correct procedures on all the donors during the remainder of the day.

On the third trip to Savannah, Beth and Mr. Stevens again work together. On the first donor, Beth sees Mr. Stevens directing the way to the refreshment stand but not taking the patient's arm. The donor faints and bruises her head.

Questions for Discussion

1. Who is at fault in this situation—Mr. Stevens, Beth, Beth's supervisor, or Mr. Stevens' supervisor?

2. If you were Beth, what would you have done differently?

3. How do you ensure proper and desired performance from someone such as a volunteer if you do not have direct management responsibility?

THE OLD-FASHIONED WAY

"I just know it will work better than the way it does now," states Bob Amos emphatically.

"Well, it looks good on paper but I'm not sure how Mr. Bivens will react," replies Shirley.

John Bivens is a well-liked department head of the facilities unit at the New Mexico Mental Health Complex. The complex is one of the largest of its type in the world providing mental health and retardation services to approximately 3,000 clients. The facilities unit is responsible for the repair and upkeep of all buildings, equipment, and grounds. Several years ago, Mr. Bivens organized the unit as indicated in Figure 12.1.

Prior to his arrival, the situation in this unit was quite bad with repair and maintenance work being performed shoddily. The work was typically performed much later than desired and many times had to be repeated because of improper procedures. Most people in the complex appear generally pleased with the work of the unit, and the credit can be primarily attributed to John Bivens. Prior to arriving at the complex, he had spent 20 years in the military in a similar role, and he had implemented many similar rules and procedures used in the military in the present setting. It is on this last point that Bob and Shirley were pursuing their conversation.

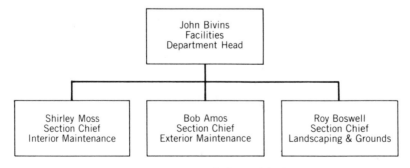

Figure 12.1. Organizational chart of facilities unit.

Several years ago Mr. Bivens had initiated a work request process that involved five forms and three signatures. All operating units in the complex must follow the procedure whenever a work repair request is made. The procedure usually requires a two-week delay after the request has been made, before work begins, unless it is an emergency.

Bob Amos had been appointed the section chief of the exterior maintenance unit about nine months ago and is discussing a streamlined work request procedure with Shirley at lunch.

"How could he possibly disagree?" queries Bob. "The way I figure it, by cutting the number of forms to only two and the required signatures to one, I estimate the work can be completed in only half the time that it now takes. I know we don't receive many official complaints, but I hear rumblings at times about how long it takes us to get to a job."

Shirley replies: "You're probably right, but you know how Mr. Bivens likes to take credit for things. He's a likeable person but definitely likes to do things his way and also be in charge. If you are sure of your idea and don't mind running the risk, why don't you talk it over with him?"

That afternoon Bob composes the following memorandum.

TO: Mr. John Bivens, Department Head Facilities Unit
FROM: Mr. Bob Amos, Section Chief Exterior Maintenance
RE: Changed Work Request Procedures

I would like to propose that we change the procedure under which work is requested of our units. As you know, the present procedure requires five forms and three signatures. I have designed a new procedure that uses only two forms and one signature. This change should reduce substantially the delay between the time the work request is made and the time the work actually begins.

Furthermore, your workload should be reduced. The proposed changes involve the section chiefs more in decision making and do not require as much involvement in the signing of papers as the present procedure. I would be happy to discuss this item with you at your convenience.

Two days later, Bob receives the following memorandum.

TO: Mr. Bob Amos, Section Chief Exterior Maintenance
FROM: Mr. John Bivens, Department Head Facilities Unit
RE: Denial of Change in Work Request Procedure

I appreciate your recent communication regarding changes in our work request procedures. We need fresh ideas in this organization and I can tell we made the correct decision when you were moved into the section chief's slot a short time ago.

However, in this instance, I see no reason to change the procedure. The procedure has worked well for many years and I see no strong reason to run the risk of ruining a good thing.

Keep up your good work.

Questions for Discussion

1. Assuming that Bob anticipated some resistance to his proposed change, what approach should he have used with Mr. Bivins?
2. Now that your proposal has been rejected, list the alternatives available to you. What would you do?

THE FISH STORY

"How many of you have ever been to Marineland, Sea World, or to one of those places where you see whales and porpoises performing?" asked the workshop facilitator.

Beverly Greene raised her hand as did most of the approximately 25 people attending a "Basic Management for Health Care Officials" workshop in New Orleans. This is the last day of a four-day workshop. Beverly has recently been appointed to be the program director in the mental health unit in a large metropolitan city health department. She is responsible for 12 people who are involved in several clinics held weekly in various parts of the city.

The leader of the workshop, Bob Bowen, is discussing employee development as he continues with his story. "In one of the most popular acts in those shows, a porpoise swims quickly along the bottom of the pool, leaps high out of the water, and goes over a rod that must be 10 feet out of the water. How many of you have seen that?" asked Bob. Again, many hands went up.

"How do you think they get those porpoises jumping 10 feet out of the water?" queried Bob.

Comments from the group included: "They train them." "They practice."

"No," Bob answered "That's not how they do it. They go out into the ocean and get on a microphone. Then they put out an invitation. 'All you porpoises who can jump 10 feet out of the water, come on over. Good career opportunities.' That's how it's done. Right?"

Beverly and the others know that Bob is teasing them to make a point.

"You know I'm kidding, but think about the process that is followed to get the porpoise to jump 10 feet out of the water. They go out into the ocean and obtain a good, average, rather normal porpoise. Then what happens?" asked Bob in a rhetorical manner. "They put the rod literally on the bottom of the pool. While the porpoise swims around the pool, nothing happens until the porpoise swims over the rod and then what happens, Jane?" asked Bob, inviting her to respond. (Jane is another participant in the workshop.)

"I guess they give the porpoise a piece of meat or something," replied Jane.

"Right," said Bob, as he seemed to become more excited as he continued with his story. "They reward the porpoise. Are we finished? No, we're not finished. We raise the rod. The porpoise swims over the raised rod and here we are with a reward again. The process continues until we have the porpoises jumping the desired 10 feet out of the water."

"Now, let's look at this process a little more seriously," Bob continued. "Admittedly this story came from the animal world, but what is so different about finding yourself a good, average, rather normal person? You work with that person and set some realistic goals that may be quite low initially. When you observe the person performing rather close to the desired goal, you give a reward. You'll notice I said 'rather close' and not perfect. Next, we raise the goals and after a period of time, if you handle it properly, you'll have your own 'porpoises' or people jumping 10 feet out of the water."

Later that evening, Beverly is continuing to reflect on the porpoise example. It is such a simple little story but seems to make sense. Set goals. Rewards. Raise goals. It does not seem to be anymore complicated than that.

That night Beverly and Jane have dinner together before catching their return flights. "How did you enjoy the workshop?" asked Jane, when she arrived at the table where Beverly was already sitting.

"It was a good experience," Beverly answered. "My degree is in counseling and I have not had much experience or training in management. I will be able to use the information when I return to work."

"I agree." Jane responded. The material was good. I hope we can attend some follow-up programs on these topics. What was your favorite session?"

"My favorite, yet most intimidating session was the one in which Bob described the porpoise story," replied Beverly.

"Yes, that was a good example, but what do you mean favorite but intimidating?" asked a confused Jane.

"I mean that the story made so much sense and I want to give it a try, but I'm not sure I know how to do it," volunteered Beverly. "My people just seem so different. Using Bob's example, it seems like some are just barely swimming at all and others might—just might—be interested in jumping a little higher! I'm also wondering about the rewards. Bob talked so much about the importance of rewards and yet the bureaucracy takes care of that. They tell us when and who we can promote. We all receive the standard percentage salary increase yearly. Even titles are prescribed by the bureaucracy."

"It does sound more complicated than it did in the workshop," responded Jane.*

Questions for Discussion

1. Discuss the advice that you would provide Beverly on the following two issues:
   a. How do you implement the "porpoise" process when people are so different?
   b. How do you administer rewards when many of them might be controlled by the 'system'?

A similar tale can be found in Blanchard, K., & Johnson, S. *The One Minute Manager*. New York: Morrow, 1982, pp. 79–81.

2. Do we need to have all our people jumping "10 feet out of the water?"

3. Suppose you believe in the goal-setting process described in the incident and you want your supervisor to use this process with you. In other words, assume the role of the "porpoise" and describe what you would do to convince your supervisor that you can "jump a little higher."

TV WATCHING IS DANGEROUS TO YOUR HEALTH

Today seems to be the most hectic day that Kay can recall in her eight years of nursing experience. Kay Dohn is the head nurse of a medical-surgical unit in City Hospital. She graduated eight years ago with a B.S. in Nursing and has worked only at City Hospital. Prior to becoming head nurse about two years ago, she had been a staff nurse and charge nurse in medical-surgical units.

One factor associated with today's chaos is that every bed in the unit except one is filled. In addition, one staff RN in Kay's unit is attending an infection control seminar and this leaves her a short-handed even though Kay knew of the program and approved the attendance. Also, about mid-morning, one of the nursing assistants received a call about her sick child and had to leave.

Kay feels as though the whole world is coming down on her and calls the nursing supervisor. "Joan, we're really running ragged up here. Nearly every bed is filled. Cathy is at the seminar. Mrs. Bowen had to go home. Do you think we could call someone in or let someone float to this unit?" inquired a desperate Kay.

"I thought things must be rough up there," replied Joan. Joan Brown is the 7–3 nursing supervisor at City Hospital. "I'll see what we can do."

Kay knows that at least for today she is not managing. She is assuming some of the patient load herself to try and ease the burden on everyone else.

Kay and all the others have been working at this pace for several hours and she has just about caught up. She sits down at the nurses' station, but 30 seconds later she sees the light go on for one of the patients.

"Yes, Mrs. Pickard. What do you need?" queried Kay from the nurses' station.

"Could I have something for pain?" the patient asked.

"I'll check your records and be right down," said Kay.

A few minutes later, Kay is on her way to the patient who has requested the medication and she thinks she recognizes some voices in a patient's room. Kay knows that the room is supposed to be empty so she tapps lightly on the door and enters.

To her surprise, she sees two nursing aides and one laboratory technician casually chatting and watching television. This behavior is in direct opposition to hospital policy and everyone is aware of the policy. Kay is even more upset because it is occurring when they are so busy in the unit.

When Kay asks the three what is happening, a consensus reply seems to be something like the following: "I just came in." "I was not watching TV." "I haven't been here long."

All three people are sent back to their jobs and Kay notifies the nursing department manager and the laboratory department manager.

In accordance with personnel policy on matters such as this situation, documentation and interviews are held. The personnel policy also provides for punishment if warranted. The laboratory technician receives three days immediate suspension without pay and has the incident placed in his personnel file. Each of the two nursing aides receives one day suspension without pay to be accomplished at a time when convenient to staffing. They also receive incidents in their personnel file.

Kay later learns, however, that the laboratory technician had just stepped in to the room and yet he received the most severe punishment.

Questions for Discussion

1. Would you have reported these three people as Kay did or would you have handled the situation differently?
2. Does the issue of fairness matter when you are involved with two different departments? In other words, how far can you carry fairness? Within departments? Between departments? Between hospitals? Between the hospital and some other employer?
3. Do you think you need a policy or procedure for each type of situation like this or a more general one that covers all professional conduct?

THE PURPOSE OF POLICIES

Sarah Renfroe had spent several years working in various positions in the North Carolina Department of Public Health. About seven months ago, she was offered the position of supervisor of the accounts payable section in the accounting department. She accepted the position and this was her first supervisory role. Eighteen people report directly to her, but she has two people she looks to as lead people even though their titles, salaries, and other benefits are not associated with these quasi-supervisory roles.

Aaron Flowers is one of the people who reports to Sarah. He is an accounting clerk who has been with the department about five months. Sarah likes Aaron because he always performs at an above-average level and is also well liked by his co-workers.

One day, he knocked on her door and said: "May I see you for just a minute, Mrs. Renfroe?"

"Sure, come on in, Aaron," replied Sarah congenially. "How is everything?"

"Pretty good, I guess. I don't have any problems here, but I do have a personal problem. My wife needs an operation that will not be covered by the health insurance and I need to borrow $500 from the credit union," Aaron explained. "Would you mind signing my application blank so I can join the credit union and borrow the money?"

"Certainly. I hope your wife does O.K.," replied Sarah, as she signs the form.

Aaron left her office and dropped the application in the departmental mail for delivery to the credit union. The department had a credit union that made loans of less than $1,000.

Three days later, Aaron returns to Sarah's office in a rather disturbed state. He starts the conversation by saying, ''I can't believe it. They turned down my request for a loan because I'm not a permanent employee. I had no idea this would happen. No one ever told me about this. Besides, what difference does it make?''

After listening to Aaron, Sarah realizes that the credit union has a policy in which only permanent employees can obtain loans. The department has a probationary period of six months and, unless someone takes action to stop it, the permanent status becomes effective the first day after the six-month period.

Sarah tried to settle Aaron down and said: ''Don't give up just yet. Give me a little time to look into the situation.''

After Aaron leaves, Sarah checks the departmental policy manual, which is rather clear on the requirement for permanent status. She then calls the supervisor of the credit union and explains that Aaron has less than one month to go before achieving permanent status. Furthermore, there is absolutely no doubt but that it would be granted because his work is excellent. She is told that the only way to make an exception to the policy would be to have the credit union board of directors approve a policy change, but it will not be meeting until the following month.

Sarah feels as though that approach will probably not work and besides Aaron needs the money now and not next month.

She decides to try another route and checks with the personnel office to see if permanent status can be granted before six months. She is told that it has never been done and there are no provisions to allow it to be done. The next meeting of the personnel system board of directors who could authorize such an exception is more than two months away.

Sarah calls Aaron back that afternoon and explains that she tried but had no success. Aaron thanks her and hangs up.

The next morning, she receives the following letter:

Dear Mrs. Renfroe,
I appreciate what you tried to do for me but I don't like the way the system operates around here.

I called my father last night and know I can get a job back on his farm at least through the harvest season.

I've enjoyed working with you.
    Sincerely,
    Aaron Flowers.

Questions for Discussion

1. Since Aaron is an above-average employee, would you try to change his mind? If so, explain the tactics you would use. If not, explain why.

2. Take one side in this incident and defend it. If you think policies such as this one serve a valid purpose and organizations need them, defend this viewpoint. On the other hand, if you think policies like this one interfere with good judgment and supervision, explain why.

3. What can a supervisor do when policies and procedures such as this one are established by someone else and perhaps a change is needed?

4. Consider your own organization. Are there any rules, policies, or procedures that may have negative consequences if enforced and don't serve any real purpose?

AN UPSET PATIENT AND DOCTOR

"Mrs. Greene, Mrs. Anne Greene, 2169," came the page over the hospital intercom system. (Anne Greene is the 3–11 supervisor at Bowden Memorial Hospital.)

Anne answers the page and begins talking by telephone with Sue Amos in the admitting office. "Mrs. Greene, Dr. Kirby just called and is upset about his patient, Mr. Bowen. Mr. Bowen is scheduled for surgery in the morning and he and Dr. Kirby want a private room but none are available," states Sue. "Mr. Bowen is threatening to go home if he doesn't get a private room."

"O.K. I'll be down to admitting in just a minute," replies Anne.

"Do we have any semi-private rooms available?" queries Anne after arriving.

"Yes, we have far more semi-private rooms than the number of patients scheduled to be admitted," replies Sue.

"Why don't you place Mr. Bowen in a semi-private room and block the other bed?" asks Anne. (Bowden has followed such a procedure for years when the census count is expected to be low. The blocked bed would not be assigned to anyone else unless no semi-private rooms are available.)

"I thought about that but Mr. Battin said that we could not do that anymore. He told us that Mrs. Strong had approved the change," replies Sue. (Mr. Battin is the controller at Bowden and Mrs. Strong is the hospital administrator.)

Anne finds this change difficult to believe because Bowden has used this procedure for years and to do otherwise does not make sense. Furthermore, any changes like this are usually widely discussed in various departmental committees.

"I know it is Sunday afternoon, but why don't you call Mr. Battin at home to verify this? I'm afraid that somehow our lines of communication have been confused," suggests Anne.

Anne observes Sue calling Mr. Battin and while she only hears one side of the conversation, it is obvious that Mr. Battin tells the admitting clerk not to block the bed, which means Mr. Bowen would be assigned a semi-private room with another patient.

When Dr. Kirby hears of the decision, he transferrs Mr. Bowen to another hospital and tries to call Mrs. Strong at home. He is unable to reach her.

The next morning, Dr. Kirby visits Mrs. Strong's office. "Who decided that patients should not be placed in semi-private rooms?" he asks.

But Mrs. Strong has only recently arrived at the office and is unaware of the problem.

"Your people told me last night that you had approved a change not to block any beds in semi-private rooms when a patient requested a private room," Dr. Kirby continues in a heated tone.

"I never issued such a change and I have no idea how it originated," states a rather surprised Mrs. Strong. "I assure you I will handle the situation, and we will continue to operate under the procedure we have used for years. I'm sorry for the confusion and inconvenience."

After Dr. Kirby leaves, Mrs. Strong asks Mr. Battin and Mrs. King to come to her office. Mrs. King is the director of nursing at Bowden. At this point, she has no knowledge of the incident that occurred the day before. After describing the prior evening's events, Mrs. Strong asks Mr. Battin, "Do you know how this situation started?"

"I sure don't," replies Mr. Battin. "I never even heard of this situation until then, and I certainly didn't initiate the change myself."

"Well, for the record, we will continue to block beds in semi-private rooms as long as other semi-private rooms are available and the patient requests a private room," states Mrs. Strong.

Later that day, Anne begins telling Mrs. King about the incident involving Dr. Kirby.

"Yes, Mrs. Strong told Mr. Battin and me this morning that no changes were made in the procedure," states Mrs. King. She also admits that it is confusing that no one seems to know the source of the alleged change. She further states: "Mr. Battin seemed as uninformed about the situation as I was."

Mrs. King notices the perplexed look on Anne's face. "What's the matter, Anne?" asks Mrs. King.

"This sounds strange to me. Yesterday, when this situation developed, I had the admitting clerk call Mr. Battin at home to verify the change," Anne explains. "I can't verify that the clerk was talking to him, but I'm sure she wouldn't pretend to call him. Are you telling me that he said he had never heard of the situation?"

"That's exactly what he said this morning," replies Mrs. King. "Since I had not talked with you at that time, I did not confront him."

Later, while Mrs. King is reviewing this situation, she wonders what she should do. She can just forget about it since no apparent permanent change has been made. On the other hand, she knows that Mr. Battin had knowledge of the situation and had participated in the decision with Dr. Kirby. Is it right for him to get off the hook by claiming no prior knowledge? She also wonders about the consequences with her own nurses if it appears that she is not supporting them.

Questions for Discussion

1. What would you do if you were Mrs. King?
2. Assume the role of one person in the incident—the admitting clerk, the evening supervisor, the director of nursing, the controller, or the hospital

administrator. Discuss anything that you would have done differently in the incident.

3. What are the ethical issues involved in covering up a co-worker's incompetency or mistakes?

CONTROL AND LEADERSHIP

Jack Gordon has worked in the health care field for eighteen years. While he has had a varied career, he is presently employed at the Community Health Clinic in Des Moines, Iowa. The clinic provides a wide range of physical and mental health services. Jack is the administrative officer of the clinic and has responsibility for all personnel, accounting, and record-keeping functions. He supervises 10 people directly, because no other supervisory personnel exist in this part of the organization. The various titles of the employees in the administrative unit are indicated in Figure 12.2. Approximately 70 people work at the clinic.

Jack enjoys working with people and considers himself a participative leader. He has a record of accomplishing things by involving people in decision making and trusting them. He smiles to himself when he reads about the "new" management's proposal for a similar style. When he read the following quote in a best-selling book, he had no trouble accepting its philosophy: "Treat people like adults." He had been supervising that way for many years and knew that the approach would work.

Recently, several events caused him to reflect on the appropriateness of his participative trusting style. About two months ago he realized that the employees were inappropriately using the office copier. On several occasions, he noticed people copying recipes, cartoons, and other material that was not work related. Deciding not to overreact on such a minor issue, he merely tacked the following notice above the office copier: "Please be sure that the copies you make are work related or place 10 cents per copy in the box." Jack believes that his low-pressure approach has worked because he has seen money in the box and has not noticed any further abuse.

During the past several weeks, it appears to Jack that people are taking longer breaks and lunch periods. The clinic does not require a sign-in–sign-out procedure, and people are allowed two 15-minute breaks daily and a one hour lunch period. The breaks and lunch can be taken anytime a person prefers. Although Jack has not been using a stopwatch on employees, he notices that several people are slightly extending the specified times. At the last employee meeting, he calmly stated the following: "I'm not trying to make a mountain out of a mole hill, but I would like to remind all of you that work procedures provide for two 15-minute breaks and one hour for lunch. Since this is such a specific requirement, I doubt if there are any questions, but I would be happy to discuss any."

There were no questions and again Jack thought he had made his point without having to resort to stronger tactics.

Yesterday afternoon, when Jack was going home, he saw one of the clinic

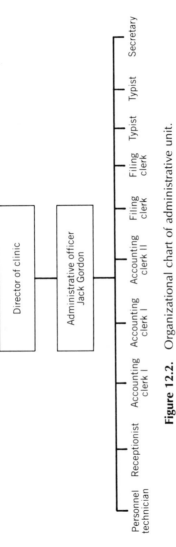

Figure 12.2. Organizational chart of administrative unit.

vehicles parked at a beer and wine package store. He noticed that one of the accounting clerks was driving the vehicle. He assumed that she had delivered some reports to the computer operations center located about five miles from the clinic, but organizational policy stipulates that vehicles are to be used for official use only, and there was no reason for the vehicle to be at the store. Jack knows that he must examine this situation further.

Questions for Discussion

1. Do you agree that Jack needs to pursue this issue further? How would you handle it?
2. Do you agree with the way he handled the copier and break situations?
3. How do you pursue the fine balance between maintaining control and yet being an effective leader? For example, technically speaking, a personal phone call is using organizational time and resources for personal use. Most supervisors do not become concerned about this kind of situation until it is abused. How do you draw the line on these cases?

"DOING IT" AND "GETTING IT DONE"

Barbara Allen had recently been appointed to be the assistant head nurse of a medical-surgical unit on the third floor of County General Hospital. County General used the assistant head nurse designation for nurses who have responsibility for shifts other than the 7 A.M.—3 P.M. shift. Barbara has responsibility for the 3 P.M.—11 P.M. shift. She had graduated from a local junior college about two years ago with an associate degree in nursing. She had worked for those two years as a staff nurse in this same medical-surgical unit and was promoted when the former Assistant Head Nurse had resigned when her husband was transferred.

When Barbara was first offered the promotion, she had some initial anxieties. Her two years at the junior college had focused almost exclusively on the technical aspects of nursing and she was unsure about the functions of an assistant head nurse position and even more unsure if she had the required skills. During her interview for the new job, she was assured by the staffing coordinator that there would be ample opportunity for her to attend management seminars and workshops and grow in her role as a manager. She remembered well the coordinator's response when she was being interviewed: "Don't worry about it. We all had to face this same situation when we were just starting in our careers. If we didn't think you could manage the unit, we wouldn't offer you this job."

Barbara has been in the new role for only a month and so far has not had any major crises. The one thing she has learned about her new leadership role, however, is that she (and other managers) must often work slightly longer than the standard eight-hour shift and also longer than when she was a staff nurse. In fact, she has come in early today so that she can finish the patient assignments for the staff nurses on her shift.

She is about two hours into the evening shift when one of her staff nurses, Mrs. Sanders, informs her that she has to leave immediately because of a sick child at the day care center. Rather than reassigning Mrs. Sanders' patients to the other staff nurses, Barbara just takes over the caseload and begins to check the medication due for the departed nurse's patients.

The evening supervisor, Mrs. Brown, is making routine rounds with a new graduate nurse and observes an improper IV chemotherapy infusion rate that the graduate nurse had initiated. After Mrs. Brown corrects the graduate nurse she tries to locate Barbara and finds her taking the 9 o'clock vital signs for Mrs. Sanders' patients. Mrs. Brown asks Barbara to be sure and see her before she leaves that evening.

Later that evening, the supervisor says: "Barbara, we are paying you to manage all the nurses and patients and not just function like a staff nurse. That situation with the new graduate nurse and the IV chemotherapy was quite serious. If you were managing the unit, you would have noticed the problem. There is a difference between 'getting it done' and 'doing it.' I know you have been in the new job only a month, but I hope you can show us more management expertise and not just nursing expertise in the future."

Barbara is too tired to respond adequately, but later, as she is driving home, she wonders what (if anything) she had done wrong and what she would do differently if a similar situation happened in the future.

Questions for Discussion

1. What alternatives were available to Barbara when the staff nurse had to leave early?
2. What response(s) should Barbara have made to the supervisor on the unit? At the post-shift conference?
3. What should Barbara's supervisor do to facilitate her (Barbara's) development as a manager?
4. How does one learn how to stop "doing it" and focus on "getting it done"?

HELPING TROUBLED EMPLOYEES

Signs of Alcohol and Drug Abuse

1. Failure to fulfill responsibilities.
2. Uncharacteristic temper tantrums.
3. Work appearance deteriorates.
4. A strong case of "alibi-itis" in explaining all problems.
5. More mistakes or errors are evident.
6. Longer lunch breaks are taken.

7. Finding employee in unusual place like storeroom, restroom, and closets more often.

8. Tardiness increases.

9. Tends to avoid people.

10. Financial difficulties emerge. (Dubrin, 1982)

After Karen Howe had read the above list, she decided to confront the situation she had with Steve Adams. She is the director of the Office of Aging, which includes 12 people in the unit, with Steve Adams as the deputy director. Steve has had an extended career in governmental health care and has performed well as the deputy director for the past three years.

During the past eight months, however Karen noticed that Steve had exhibited most of the tell-tale signs in the above list on numerous occasions. When things are going well, he is an excellent administrator. For the past several months, however, he has let things slide, and his moody behavior is causing resentment among the rest of the staff. Karen realizes that unless she confronts Steve with the problem, she is not fulfilling her role as director. She has been somewhat hesitant in the past because of the sensitivity of the issue, but the department recently initiated an Employee Assistance Program designed to help employees with personal problems and with this added support Karen knows that she must act.

Karen asks Steve to stay after normal working hours to have a private meeting. Karen tries to relax and almost immediately deals with the severity of the problem as she perceives it: "Steve, I'm concerned about your health and your work."

"What do you mean? I've had things under control and I've only missed a couple of days of work in the past year," replied Steve.

"Steve, your progress on the annual report has been below average at best and I've noticed that you're more argumentative with the other people than you were in the past," Karen said.

"Well, maybe things have slipped a little bit, but I've been under a lot of pressure lately. How serious do you see things?" asked Steve.

"Serious enough that I think you need to visit the Employee Assistance Program counselor. You recall the department recently established this program for employees with personal problems and it is my perception that your problems are personal in nature and not directly work related," Karen stated.

After continued discussion, Steve agrees to visit the counselor. He realizes that he has a drinking problem and agrees to visit the next Alcoholics Anonymous (AA) meeting. Steve joins the organization and attends meetings regularly. Karen keeps in close contact with Steve's counselor and meets with Steve for a review of his progress.

Karen asked, "Steve, how do you feel about your work and any progress on your problem?"

"I feel better. I seem to be able to concentrate more on work and I know my attitude has changed," replied Steve.

"I agree," Karen said. "Several people have told me that you seem like a new person and your work on the annual report was good. We'll continue to meet about once a month to review progress and I hope you see the benefits of the counseling program.''

''I agree that the program has helped me. I plan to continue to attend the AA meetings and I appreciate your giving me a chance. I know that everyone would not have done what you did,'' Steve replied.

About two months later, Steve is out for three days and does not call in. When she tries to reach him at home, there is no answer. After he returns to work and is asked about his absence, he replies, ''I went out and got real drunk.''

Questions for Discussion

1. State the pro and con arguments regarding programs such as these.
2. What would you do with Steve now?
3. How can you defend using organizational resources to help people with problems like alcoholism, drug abuse, and gambling?
4. Should such employees ever be fired? When?

THE LATE WORKER

Gail Hawkins is the director of the pharmacy at the Veterans Memorial Hospital in Dallas, Texas. The hospital is a 300-bed, general purpose one, and Gail has been the director for the past three years. The hospital pharmacy is open from 7 A.M. to 11 P.M. on weekdays and 7 A.M. to 1 P.M. on weekends. She supervises 11 people of whom five are registered pharmacists. The remaining six are pharmacy technicians, couriers, and clerks.

Gail is experiencing a problem with one of the clerks, Mrs. Gilbert. Mrs. Gilbert works the evening shift on weekdays and never works the weekend. She is a capable person and has seven years of experience on the job. For the past couple of months, Mrs. Gilbert has had trouble arriving at work on time. Hospital policy requires that people arrive 15 minutes early in order that any information can be exchanged as the shift changes. Gail had never noticed this problem in the past, but approximately two months ago, Mrs. Gilbert would arrive 10–15 minutes late about one day a week. Gail did not do anything at this point because no one else, including the clerk on the off-going shift, complained and Mrs. Gilbert's performance otherwise was quite satisfactory.

Last week, the other clerk, Mr. Bowman, asked to talk with Gail.

''Come on in, Mr. Bowman. What's on your mind?'' asked Gail.

''Oh, not too much,'' responded Mr. Bowman. ''Do you mind if I close this door?''

After the door was closed and Mr. Bowman had taken a chair, he seemed reluctant to talk.

Gail asked him, "You seem ill at ease, Mr. Bowman. What's the problem?"

"Well, I just don't want to be a troublemaker. I like our pharmacy unit here and in general we all work well together. My problem is with Mrs. Gilbert. For the last two weeks she has been 15 minutes late three days each week. Ordinarily, I would not be too upset about this, but I have to pick up my child from school at 3:15 P.M., and I have to leave here on time or I never make it," said Mr. Bowman.

"I didn't know this was happening. We've been having so many department head meetings lately on our new organizational plan that I have not been here during shift changes," replied Gail. "I'll talk with her and we'll straighten things out."

The next day Mrs. Gilbert arrived on time and Gail later discussed the situation with her. Mrs. Gilbert stated that she had taken a part-time job that occasionally caused her to be a few minutes late but that she would do her best to improve.

Gail felt that Mrs. Gilbert was sincere and decided that just mentioning the situation to her was sufficient. The conversation ended on a seemingly pleasant note and both seemed to accept the discussion in a positive way.

The next day, Mrs. Gilbert seemed quite cold to Mr. Bowman as they exchanged information at shift change. The coldness continued for several days, and Mrs. Bowman confronted Mrs. Gilbert by saying: "I hope I'm not being too personal but you have seemed moody lately. Is there anything I could do to help?"

"Sure is. Stop tattling. That's what you can do," replied Mrs. Gilbert angrily.

"I'm not sure I know what you mean," stated a somewhat surprised Mr. Bowman.

"I'm sure you do know. You went and told Dr. Hawkins that I have been coming to work late. How about all those times I came in early? Did you tell her about those?" challenged Mrs. Gilbert.

"Listen, I didn't mean to cause any problems, but I have to pick up my child from school at 3:15 and I need to leave here by 3 o'clock," said Mr. Bowman.

A few more words were exchanged with Mrs. Gilbert being reasonably hostile and Mr. Bowman trying to explain his rationale for talking with Gail.

The next day Gail asked Mr. Bowman how things were between him and Mrs. Gilbert.

"I don't see any major problems. I think everything will work out fine," he replied. He does not really feel this way because the relationship between the two is tense but he is reluctant to say anything because he does not want to cause anyone trouble and Mrs. Gilbert had reacted so negatively before.

For the next several weeks, Gail pays closer attention to the situation and Mrs. Gilbert shows up on time on every occasion. One day, Mr. Bowman approached Gail and said, "I really don't know what to do, but Mrs. Gilbert and I are not working well together. I fibbed a little bit—no alot—when you asked me how things were. She has been cold since I talked with you and accused me of tattling. For the past week, she has been leaving me work from her shift, which means I have to do mine plus some of hers. If this keeps up, I still won't be able to make it to school on time. Can you tell me what to do to avoid making things even worse between us?"

Questions for Discussion

1. What would you say to Mr. Bowman at this point?
2. How would you resolve the conflict?
3. Assume Gail Hawkin's role. Did she handle the situation properly, or would you have handled things differently?

WHAT NEEDS ENRICHING?

John Wilson became more depressed as he read the responses before him:

Enrich my pocketbook. That's what needs enriching.

I'm too old to get excited about another new management fad.

f we're being asked to take on more responsibility, where is the added reward? If I stick my neck out further by taking on more challenges, all that means is there is more room to cut my throat.

I'm not sure our union agrees with job enrichment. I'll need to see how they react before I can give a commitment.

Nearly all the responses John read expressed concerns similar to those above. John is the supervisor of the physical therapy unit at a large regional hospital in the southwestern United States. He supervises 16 people who are divided into three sections, each having a section leader. The section leader's role is not a tremendously strong one, since John handles most of the administrative requirements. He thinks this is the best approach because he feels that all his people, including the section chiefs, prefer the "hands on" aspects of their job as opposed to the "paperwork." All of the people belong to a local union and the relations between management and union can be described as rather neutral at the moment.

The responses that he was reading are some of the employees' reactions to the discussion held last week concerning a job enrichment program. After he had explained the program to the people he had asked them to give him their anonymous replies.

He had considered job enrichment because the morale in his unit had become quite low and he has had three recent resignations. After reading about job enrichment, he had described it to his people as a way to provide them more challenging, responsible jobs. According to what he had read, if properly administered, job enrichment could lead to higher performance and morale and less absenteeism and turnover. He explained to his people that more variety, autonomy, feedback, and significance would be built into their jobs. These factors were more or less the "ingredients" of an enriched job.

He recalls from his explanation that few questions were asked at the time. He also remembers that someone asked what it would mean to have more autonomy. He replied that one example might concern the schedule. Whereas John presently made out the schedules for everyone, he could let the section chiefs be involved or might even allow employees to sign up for various parts of the schedule. He also remembers a difficult question that someone raised about his own role (John's) after the enrichment. The question was something as follows: "If we will be doing the things that you have been doing, what will you do?" John admits now that his response to this question was probably weak and rather vague.

John is perplexed concerning what his next set of steps should be. He has undertaken the job enrichment idea on his own, and as far as he knows, no one else in the hospital is doing anything similar. He had not felt it necessary to receive any kind of approval because he had not anticipated any major changes or resource requirements. He assumed that people would merely perform their work differently.

Questions for Disscussion

1. Often we hear of similar employee reactions when managers try new ideas, such as quality control circles, MBO (management by objectives), and job enrichment. What can be done to lessen the negative reactions to change?
2. In John's specific case, do you think job enrichment was an appropriate tool? If so, how would you have approached it? If not, what would you propose doing about the low morale and turnover problem?
3. Do you think he should have sought some higher approval before he tried to implement job enrichment?

REDUCTION IN STAFF (A)

"You seem a bit edgy tonight," commented Bob Greene to his wife Sally as they were enjoying an evening meal at one of Seattle's finest restaurants.

"Well, I'm trying not to be," responded Sally. "I know I try not to bring my work home with me and I didn't actually bring any home, except up here," she said, pointing to her head.

"What's the problem? I'll be your resident psychiatrist," Bob said, trying to relieve some of Sally's apparent tension.

"There are actually two related concerns. I don't think I told you but we received some information from Washington last week, which means that we will have to cut back on programs," said Sally. Sally is the project director of a pilot program funded directly by the federal government. The funds are administered through the state's Division of Children's Programs. The program is experimental and is the only one of its kind. She supervises 20 people who are formed into teams of four, and each team holds drug abuse counseling clinics three days a week in various parts of Seattle. The program has been funded for three years, and Sally was hired as the first project director 10 months ago. The correspondence from Washington requires a 15 percent reduction in the personnel budget for the second year of the project, which starts two months from now. The particular way to achieve the reduction was not specified. It might involve laying off 15 percent of the present employees, or requiring all present employees to take a 15 percent cut, or anything else as long as a total personnel budget is reduced by 15 percent.

"The actual layoff is certainly one problem and I hate to deal with it. That's one unpleasant part about supervision. All the people in the unit are good and I don't like to think about the impact on families and others when a person loses a job," responded Sally. "The other problem I have is how to achieve the 15 percent reduction. I was reading an article in a journal on leadership and the author said that, despite all the research conducted on leadership, a decision maker essentially had three choices. The leader could make the decision without any employee input. The employees could be consulted before the decision, but the leader would still make the final decision. The third approach would involve the leader giving the problem to the group after defining the limits of the decision."

Bob responded, "I never really thought about it like that. In other words, you could just announce the reduction, 'I have decided that this is the way we'll achieve the reduction, or something like that?"

"Yes, something like that," Sally replied.

"You could talk with your team leaders or all the people for that matter and receive their ideas and sentiments and then decide. Correct?" queried Bob.

"That's about it. In the third situation, I would say something like, 'as long as we reduce the personnel budget by 15 percent and have a reduction that is accepted as a fair one, I really don't care specifically what we do,'" concluded Sally.

"At least I see the two problems you have. Let's finish our dinner and enjoy the rest of the evening," said Bob.

Questions for Discussion

1. For the three leadership styles—autocratic, consultative, and group based—describe decision-making situations in which a particular style is more appropriate. In other words, what are some situations in which the autocratic approach to decision making is the more appropriate one? The consultative style? The group-based style?
2. Which approach do you think is the best choice here? Explain why.
3. It has been said that the choice of a leadership style depends on the leader, the led, and the situation. What are some additional factors associated with these three rather general ones?

REDUCTION IN STAFF (B)

Sally Greene is the project director of a federally funded program designed to offer drug abuse counseling services. Sally is faced with the problem of achieving a 15 percent reduction in the personnel budget for the upcoming fiscal year. The cut has been mandated by the federal government and would have to be implemented in about two months. Sally supervises 20 people who are divided into teams of four, with one person being designated as team leader. Although the teams are alike in structure, each team provides services in different locations in the city.

Having heard so much about the merits of participative and consultative leadership, she decides to involve the five team leaders in decision making.

After Sally had explained the background of the problem, she asked for suggestions. "Now that you've heard the problem, what do you think we should do?"

"Do I understand it correctly that it doesn't matter how we achieve the 15 percent reduction in salaries?" asked Faye Robbins. "Let's see, 15 percent multiplied by 20 people. That's about 3 people if each person's salary was the same. In other words, we don't actually have to lay off 3 people."

"That's correct. We can use any approach we want and that's why I thought together we could explore more possibilities in order to find the best approach," Sally replied.

"Before we jump right into it, are there any other tactics we could use?" asked Beverly Adams. "For example, do you think we could request a postponement or write up a report on the negative impact that the cutback will have?"

"No. The message we received was rather clear. Be prepared for a 15 percent reduction in personnel budgets in 60 days," stated Sally. "Let's see if we can name some options. George, what do you recommend?"

"I'm not sure I'd recommend it, but let's just call it an option," responded George Bivins, one of Sally's most capable team leaders. "We could require everyone to take a 15 percent cut in salary. While no one would be particularly happy about it, at least no one would lose a job."

"I'm glad you didn't recommend that one," replied Jan Jones eagerly. "While all our people are generally pretty good, some are better than others. I think we would be sending the wrong signal to the above-average performers if we cut their salaries also. We should reduce the salaries of the below-average performers or let enought of them go to reach the required reduction."

"That's what 1 was thinking when I volunteered it as an option. Besides, I wouldn't be too happy with having my salary reduced," said George. "I don't think as team leaders we should face the same cuts as everyone else."

"We would have to handle that at some point. Let's move on and receive other proposals. Anne, we haven't heard from you yet. What do you think?"

"I don't like either one that I've heard so far. I think seniority counts. While none of us have been with the project an extremely long time, some of us have been here since the beginning. I think the last ones hired should be the first to go," contributed Anne.

"All right. We have three proposals at this stage. George suggested an across-the-board 15 percent decrease, Jan wanted to base the reduction on performance, and Anne wanted to use reverse seniority," summarized Sally. "Can you think of others?"

Questions for Discussion

1. Answer Sally's last question. Are there other alternatives available?
2. What should Sally's actions be from this point forward? In other words, after all the alternatives have been identified, what should she do to achieve a consensus on the preferred alternative?
3. In hindsight, what did Sally do to facilitate the decision-making process. What should she have done differently?

REFERENCES

DuBrin, A. J. *Contemporary Applied Management*. Plano, TX: Business Publications, 1982.

Flippo, E. B., & Munsinger, G. M. *Management*. Boston: Allyn & Bacon, 1982.

Griffin, R. W. *Management*. Boston: Houghton Mifflin, 1984.

Huse, E. F. *Management*. St. Paul: West, 1982.

Kramer, M., & Schmalenberg, C. (1976, October). "Conflict: The cutting edge of growth." *Journal of Nursing Administration*, 21–23.

Naisbitt, J. *Megatrends*. New York: Warner Books, 1982.

Robbins, S. P. *Management: Concepts and Practices*. Englewood Cliffs, NJ: Prentice-Hall, 1984.

Robbins, S. P. *Managing Organizational Conflict: A Nontraditional Approach*. Englewood Cliffs, NJ: Prentice-Hall, 1974.

Schermerhorn, J. R. *Management for Productivity*. New York: Wiley, 1984.

Thomas, K. W., & Schmidt, W. H. (1976, June). "A survey of managerial interests with respect to conflict." *Academy of Management Journal*, 315–318.

Chapter Thirteen

Health Care Ethics

The field of health care is confronted with almost endless ethical considerations in today's highly technological and advancing society. Because of significant advances made in medical technology and procedures, it has been said that we are living in a "biological revolution" (Kieffer, 1979, p.1). Consider, for example, the following questions that only a few years ago were rarely discussed or debated (Kieffer, 1979):

- Should defective fetuses be aborted?
- Will only people who can afford life-prolonging and expensive medical care be treated?
- Do we as a nation of affluence have the right to dictate population policy to less-wealthy nations?
- Do we have any moral obligations to those yet unborn?

We could continue but the point is that our society today faces significant ethical issues and many of these are associated with health care decision making.

Our purpose in this chapter is not to address specific issues such as abortion, death and dying, or contraception methods. Rather, we hope to present a perspective toward ethical thinking and to provide guidelines for increasing the likelihood of ethical actions as decisions are made.

DEFINITION OF TERMS

Several terms that will be used in this chapter are defined as follows:

- *Ethics*—The system or code of morals or of a particular person, religion, group, or profession (Schermerhorn, 1984).

- *Moral*—Relating to, dealing with, or capable of making distinctions between right and wrong in conduct; good or right in conduct or character (Schermerhorn, 1984).
- *Ethical*—Having to do with ethics or morality; of or conforming to moral standards; conforming to the standards of conduct of a particular profession or group (Schermerhorn, 1984).
- *Values*—Generalized concepts of the desirable (Kieffer, 1979).
- *Teleological ethics*—An approach to ethical decision making that judges the rightness or wrongness of a particular act by the end result or consequence of a particular choice (Greer, 1983).
- *Imperative ethics*—An approach to ethical decision making that holds actions morally correct or incorrect in and of themselves regardless of the outcome or consequence; For example, "Lying is always wrong, no matter what the consequences" (Greer, 1983).

A SUPERVISORY PERSPECTIVE TOWARD ETHICS

Ethical behavior has been defined as behavior that fully encompasses legal behavior plus "something else" (Schermerhorn, 1984). In Figure 13.1, we see in the upper portion quite a distance between legal and illegal acts. In other words, one might say the following: "We didn't even come close to breaking the law." In the lower portion of the figure, we see that we barely avoided committing an illegal act, and the ethical dimension of the decision has been significantly reduced as reflected in the much shorter line.

Consider the following hypothetical examples that illustrate this point:

- *Case 1:* One of your employees takes home a half-used wooden pencil and uses it on work-related materials.
- *Case 2:* Same situation as above, except this employee gives the half-used pencil to a child at home so that the child's schoolwork can be completed.
- *Case 3:* Same employee takes home one new wooden pencil and uses it for personal correspondence.
- *Case 4:* Two wooden pencils—valued at 15 cents—are taken home by the same employee.
- *Case 5:* Employee takes home a package of 12 wooden pencils—valued at one dollar—and gives the pencils to orphans at a local orphanage.
- *Case 6:* The employee takes home a package of 12 pencils and gives them to a family member as a gift.
- *Case 7:* The employee sells the pencils for 75 cents.
- *Case 8:* The employee takes home a case—72 dozen pencils—that will be sold and the money pocketed for personal use.

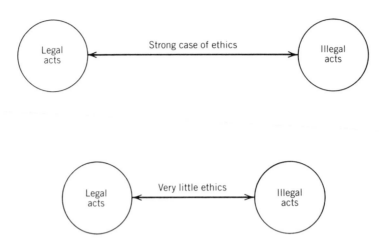

Figure 13.1. Ethics, legal, and illegal acts.

In the first situation, most supervisors probably would have little concern about the employee taking a company pencil. The distinction between a legal act and an illegal act is quite clear. Probably no one would make an issue of the first situation because no law was broken even though technically a company asset was removed from the premises. In the eighth case—and possibly others—the distinction between a legal act and an illegal one has become blurred, and many supervisors probably would consider the last case a situation of theft and consequently an illegal act. The ethical dilemma that the supervisor faces is, "Where do you draw the line?" In the cases above, where have we moved from completely ethical acts, to unethical yet legal acts, to illegal acts? The answer partially depends on the philosophical basis through which the decision maker approaches a particular situation.

There are two basic approaches for assessing the rightness or wrongness of a particular act. The teleological or consequentalist approach specifies that the "rightness or wrongness of an action is determined solely by the results of the action" (Kieffer, 1979, p. 53). This philosophy could justify an act as right under a particular set of circumstances. Rather than declare an act right or wrong, this school of thought would decide based on an "it all depends" perspective. In the pencil examples above, the donation of the pencils to orphans could make the action a proper one, whereas the selling of the pencils might be assessed as an improper one.

The opposing viewpoint—imperative ethics—judges actions in and of themselves. This perspective is more definite because yes–no responses are provided, rather than "it all depends." For example, the imperative thinker, believing that lying is wrong—always wrong, would not consider it an appropriate action if a nurse "lied" to the child to postpone the agony of the loss of parents in an automobile accident. An imperative thinker would believe that abortion and the curtailment of life support systems would constitute murder regardless of circumstances.

Table 13.1

Personal	Reference Group	Organization	Society
Values	What "they" do and say	Rules and Norms	Laws
Family	Rewards/punishment "they"	What kind of behavior is	Values
Tradition	receive as result of behavior	supported	Pressures
Religion		Policies and Procedures	Laxity/Firmness

Another factor that influences a person's decision regarding a proper and improper decision is the particular set of values that the person possesses. Values of honesty, fairness, responsibility, kindness, and equality are possessed by all but in varying degrees. Some people, of course, are more honest than others. The extent to which a person has a strong sense of positive values would influence the particular action taken in a specific situation.

FACTORS AFFECTING SUPERVISORY ETHICS

Ethics constitute the "grey area" between the rightness and wrongness of decision making. In a classic *Harvard Business Review* article, 1,200 executives responded that such things as publicity, public awareness and consciousness, societal pressures, education of managers, and governmental regulation led to higher standards of ethical conduct (Brenner & Hollander, 1977). Competition, social decay, permissive society, selfishness, and worship of the dollar as a measure of success were among the factors cited as causing lower standards of ethical behavior.

Table 13.1 categorizes these influences and shows how ethical or unethical behavior results. We can see that multiple facets impact on an individual as he or she approaches a particular situation that has degrees of rightness or wrongness associated with various alternative decisions.

A QUESTIONING APPROACH TO ETHICS

Because of the "grey area" referred to earlier, it is difficult to specify a precise model or set of steps to be followed toward making more ethical decisions. Rather, through a series of questions, we will highlight some of the issues a supervisor should consider as decisions are made. The list of questions is not comprehensive, however, nor are the questions prioritized. By examining the questions, a supervisor should be more sensitive to the concern for ethical decision making and that sensitivity should be reflected in decisions exhibiting a stronger ethical foundation.

1. Can I Live with the Decision or Action I Am About To Pursue?

We earlier showed how personal factors enter into the ethics of decision making. Certainly, different people will react differently when confronted with similar situations because of these personal differences. The implication of this question suggests that if the decision maker feels uneasy, guilty, or awkward in taking a certain action, there is probably a lack of appropriate ethics involved. Suppose you are a nurse manager in a hospital and you know that one of your peers has made a medication error. The error has already been made and the patient suffered no negative consequences. There is no way that the physician nor anyone else will ever know unless you reveal the error. You are tempted to not reveal the mistake but you remember that this same person who made the mistake has been placed on probation for two earlier medication mistakes. A third medication mistake will lead to dismissal of the employee. You decide to not reveal the error but your conscience bothers you. What we are suggesting is that actions be taken, which do not later cause such uneasiness or quesions of conscience.

2. Would I Want Those Close to Me to Know of the Action I Have Taken?

Each person has various reference groups, such as family, friends, neighbors, and co-workers. Could I ''hold my head up high'' and be proud of the decision I made or would I hope that no one close to me found out? If I anticipate embarrassment or ridicule if my action becomes known, I probably need to reconsider the ethical dimensions of my proposed decision.

3. Would I Want My Employees to Do the Same?

Suppose that you decide to use the company telephone to make a long distance call to a friend whom you are planning to visit on vacation this summer. The call is for strictly personal reasons. You rationalize your action by estimating that the call will cost only two dollars and the company owes you that much because you had to drive your car locally on business and were not reimbursed. While you may be able to ''live with this'' decision because of your rationalization and you will not be embarrassed if those close to you found out, would such actions taken by those who work in the unit you supervise seem just as rational to you? Setting the proper example is a sound basis for more ethical decisions.

4. Have I Thought about the Long-run and the Total Costs Involved?

The long-run perspective probably does not need a definition, but we should consider the eventual consequences of an action and not just what is expedient in the short run. The Lockheed Corporation justified bribes paid to foreign officials because American jobs were at stake. This short-run perspective did not consider the long-run consequences of loss of image by the corporation when the actions were revealed, potential fines and jail sentences given to guilty officials, and administrative time involved in explaining the actions. A questioning attitude that attempts to consider the multiple and continuing consequences to a proposed action will be helpful.

The *total costs* perspective is somewhat related to the long-run consideration, but is different at the same time. *Total costs* has little to do with the accounting and economic interest in fixed and variable costs, instead, *total costs* means *all* the costs involved in a particular decision. At times, we make improper and unethical decisions when we fail to consider *all* the costs. Earlier in this chapter, we presented a series of cases concerning an employee taking pencils from the company. Suppose that after taking one dozen pencils, you assess the cost as being only one dollar. This assessment is far too narrow for a total costs perspective. In addition to the one-dollar direct cost, there are potential costs associated with the following:

1. What if other employees see me doing this and assume that it is proper for them to do the same?
2. What if my supervisor finds out and I have to spend my time and his or hers explaining my action?
3. What if the company decides to make an issue out of my action and terminates my employment?
4. What has it cost if I fall in stature in the eyes of those I supervise?

The list could go on, but it is important to consider *all* the likely or unlikely costs involved in making a certain choice.

5. What Are the Multiple Viewpoints Involved?

In several of the examples above, we allowed the decision maker to defend the action taken through a rationalization process. The focus of this question involves whether others, such as those shown in Figure 13.2, would rationalize the action in the same way. Your action made good sense to you and was completely defendable. If others would react in the same way, you probably made an ethical decision.

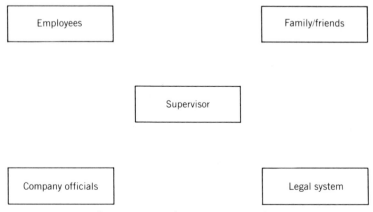

Figure 13.2. Alternative viewpoints.

6. Who Will Be Hurt by My Action?

Consider the various people or groups that could potentially be negatively impacted by a certain decision that could be interpreted as unethical:

- Self
- Family and friends
- Co-workers
- Employing organization
- Society in general

Some kinds of decisions have broader impact than others. For example, suppose you use the company telephone for personal business. You talk for less than one minute on a local call. Is such a call unethical? Most people would probably say "no" because, even though the company is "hurt" since you could have been working during that time, the "hurt" is rather insignificant. On the other hand, who is "hurt" if you fail to report a worker who performed an unsafe, yet legal procedure? You may be "hurting" yourself, if your coverup is discovered or if you feel guilty because of your silence. You may "hurt" the person guilty of the offense by not allowing the person to receive corrective instruction. You may "hurt" the person on whom the unsafe procedure was performed if there are negative consequences. You may "hurt" your employer through loss of image and potential costs of litigation. It may seem simple, but if you can say that no one is "hurt" by your action, you are probably making an ethical choice.

7. What Values (or Lack of Values) Are Reflected in My Decision?

We earlier mentioned the role that traditional values, such as fairness, honesty, and kindness, play in influencing the final choice made. As you consider what action you should take in a particular situation, it should be proven helpful to ask a question using each value as a base. For example, how honest is my contemplated act? How fair would my action be to all parties involved?

8. What Is My Motive in the Proposed Decision?

At times, determining the motive of a contemplated act can be of assistance in deciding on the more ethical choice. We earlier described a situation in which a co-worker followed an improper procedure in the delivery of health care. Consider the following motives that one might have in trying to decide whether to report the incident:

1. The interest in reporting the incident might be to just "hurt" the other person because that person is not liked.
2. The motive might be in "getting even" because the employee guilty of the infraction reported someone else in the past.

3. The motive might be to help the employee receive the necessary training or assistance so that similar situations can be avoided.

4. The concern might be trying to stem lawsuits and negative public relations associated with a later discovery of the incident.

Although there could be other motives, it can be seen that some of the motives reflect a positive concern while others are more negative. Actions pursued for positive reasons can be more easily defended and justified than those undertaken merely to inflict pain, embarrassment, or ridicule.

9. What Is the Distance Between a Completely Legal and Completely Illegal Action?

We earlier stated that ethics is the ingredient that separated legal acts from illegal acts. Let us return to our eight case situations in which the employee took home pencils. In the first case—taking home a half-used pencil for company related work—the act was totally legal and most people would say ethical. In the last case—taking a case of pencils and selling them for personal gain—a theft has occurred and obviously we are in an illegal act situation. It would be helpful as you face ethical dilemmas to reflect on this distance concept and ask yourself the question: If I undertake the action I am considering, how close have I come to an illegal act? As the distance between completely legal and completely illegal acts is reduced, the acts are becoming more and more unethical.

10. Why Should You or Why Should You Not Take a Proposed Action?

After reflecting on the series of questions proposed here, it would be helpful to list the reasons why you should take a certain action and then list why you should not. If you are honest with yourself and objective, the listing should point the way to the more preferred act.

These ten questions are not intended to be ironclad, theoretically derived models

Table 13.2

1. Can I live with the decision or action I am about to pursue?
2. Would I want those close to me to know of the action I have taken?
3. Would I want my employees to do the same?
4. Have I thought about the long run and the total costs involved?
5. What are the multiple viewpoints involved?
6. Who will be hurt by my action?
7. What values (or lack of values) are reflected in my decision?
8. What is my motive in the proposed decision?
9. What is the distance between a completely legal and completely illegal action?
10. Why should you or why should you not take a proposed action?

to be used in supervisory decision making. Rather, the listing is intended to sensitize the supervisor to the kinds of issues that should be considered. Table 13.2 summarizes these issues.

THE ROLE OF THE SUPERVISOR IN ETHICAL ISSUES

An extended research study attempted to determine the causes of ethical and unethical behavior (Baumhart, 1961). The ranked responses of the managers surveyed showed that a personal code of ethics, behavior of supervisors, formal company policy, ethical climate of the industry, and behavior of equals in the company were the factors causing ethical behavior. The ranked causes of unethical behavior were behavior of superiors, ethical climate of industry, behavior of equals in the company, lack of company policy, and personal finances. As a supervisor, you are encouraged to reflect on the results of this study. The second most important factor contributing to ethical behavior is the behavior of superiors. The most important factor causing unethical behavior is the behavior of superiors. The message here is that supervisors are obligated to set a proper example and positively influence the actions of employees. In addition, the supervisor should attempt to ensure that reward practices do not create undue pressures, which can lead to unethical behavior.

It has been suggested that managers and supervisors look for simplified guidelines to be followed in making more ethical decisions (Davis, 1980). Two suggested guidelines are the "TV test" and the "family test." If the manager can pass both tests, the proposed decision is probably an ethical one. The "TV test" asks the following questions:

Could you explain your action on TV and have it accepted as a reasonable one by the audience?

The "family test" asks the following:

Would you feel comfortable explaining your action to your family, close friends, and loved ones?

Even though the two "tests" are rather simple each suggests values, conscience, and proper behavior, which fundamentally is all that ethics encompasses.

SUMMARY

Possibly because ethics has such a personal dimension, a considerable amount of research has not been conducted. Furthermore, we have not developed an "ethical model" that should be followed by all people in all situations. Hopefully, this chapter raised the awareness and sensitivity of supervisors toward the topic. The following list summarizes some of the more important ideas in this chapter.

- Probably more than in any other field, health care is facing numerous ethical dilemmas.
- There are benefits beyond the obvious ones of maintaining and promoting high levels of ethical conduct.
- The "distance" between legal and illegal acts can be expressed as ethics.
- Acts can be judged in terms of the consequences that occur or the acts themselves.
- Personal factors reference group behavior, and employing organizational practices and societal behavior are influences on ethical behavior.
- A questioning attitude will help to raise the level of ethical behavior.
- Supervisory behavior has a considerable influence on ethical and unethical acts.
- The "family test" and the "TV test" are simplified guidelines for ethical decision making.

REFERENCES

Baumhart. R. (1961, July/August). "How ethical are businessmen?" *Harvard Business Review,* 6.

Brenner, S. N., & Hollander, E. A. (1977, January/February). "Is the ethics of business changing?" *Harvard Business Review,* 57–71.

Davis, K., et al. *Business and Society.* New York: Macmillan, 1980.

Greer, D. F. *Business, Government, and Society.* New York: Macmillan, 1983.

Kieffer, G. F. *Bioethics: A Textbook of Issues.* Reading, MA: Addison-Wesley, 1979.

Schermerhorn, J. R. *Management for Productivity.* New York: Wiley, 1984.

Index